Quiet in Motion

How to Stay Calm and Focused While Life Moves Fast

I0112041

Not just another productivity or wellness book, this will be a practical yet spiritual (not religious) framework to help people

ISBN: 978-1-956369-23-6

Table Of Content

INTRODUCTION

Why Clarity Feels So Out of Reach - And Why It Doesn't Have to Be

Take a breath. *No, really. Right here.* Right now. In through your nose. Out through your mouth. Let the noise fall away, even if just for a moment. You made it to this page, and that's not nothing.

Because let's be honest - *you're tired.*

Not just the kind of tired that a nap or weekend getaway can fix, but soul-tired. Mentally foggy. Emotionally stretched. Spiritually cluttered.

You've probably read books before. Maybe even a few just like this one. You've tried the morning routines, the productivity hacks, the guided meditations, and the "just be grateful" advice that felt more like a dismissal than a solution.

So why read this one?

Because this time, it isn't about hustling harder or fixing yourself. It's about *coming home to yourself.*

The world is a clogged and noisy place, and most times, we are the factors that contribute to the distortions around us, victims of the effects of these distortions, or both. One of the devastating effects that the age of industrialization brought on us was concerning levels of psychological disruptions caused by the inability of the mind to keep up with everything going on all at once.

Every day, we are constantly bombarded with information from the fast-paced, ever-drifting, hyperconnected world. We grapple with everything stuffed into the brain, struggle to organize it all accordingly, and scuffle through everything that the world demands us to know all at once. All these have led to a form of mental clutter that has messed up our sense of focus, increased overall stress levels, and contributed to burnout in individuals.

You don't have to wait for the moment when that overwhelming feeling comes over you. Responding to the health demands of the body when it has gotten to its breaking point is extremely dangerous. You need to be constantly conscious of the reality that the mind always needs to take a break, and this is where we come about the journey together - the journey of a *clear mind, full life.*"

So this is not another feel-good book that will promise peace through just vision boards and bullet journals (though, if those help you - beautiful!). What you have is a clear, practical, spiritually honest invitation to return to clarity, intention, and presence even in a chaotic world.

So you should not be worried about becoming someone new. We'll be talking about remembering who you were before the world got so loud. Inside, we'll explore:

• How to declutter your inner world so you can think and feel with more clarity

• How to set boundaries without guilt

• How to use mindfulness, not as a trend, but as a lifeline

• How to design a routine that makes you feel human, not robotic

• How to journal in a way that's real, not performative

• And how to stop chasing your worth and start living your life

You can read it cover to cover, or you can jump around. You can underline, dog-ear, scribble in the margins... whichever works for you. You can stop after a paragraph and just sit with it. This is your journey. There's no wrong way to walk it.

Each chapter is short on purpose - because your attention is sacred, and within each, you'll find:

• A short reflection or story

- A tool or practice that's actually doable

- A quote or affirmation to carry with you

Don't rush. Let it soak in. Let it sit with you on hard days. Let it meet you in the in-between moments - before bed, during a lunch break, on a long walk. And together, we can make something of the whole rubble.

Like you, I'm only human, and while I wear many hats - writer, speaker, mental wellness educator - at my core, I'm someone who believes in the quiet, transformative power of clarity.

For over a decade, I've worked at the intersection of emotional wellness, mindful living, and intentional productivity. My career has taken me into therapy rooms, classrooms, corporate retreats, and community circles, all in service of one thing: helping people reconnect with themselves in a world that often pulls them apart.

I've led workshops for individuals feeling stuck. I've coached creatives navigating burnout. I've sat across from CEOs, college students, overwhelmed parents, and late-night journalers - people just like you - who want to feel present again but don't know where to begin.

But this work isn't just professional. It's personal.

I live what I teach. I'm a parent, a partner, a friend. I know the joy of slow Saturday mornings, the pull between ambition and rest, the guilt that can come with saying "no," and the courage it takes to create boundaries where none existed before.

And I've learned that healing doesn't happen in isolation. It happens in honest conversations and in simple, consistent choices that honor who we are. That's what this book is. A conversation. A companion. A collection of what I've learned through research, practice, and failure.

This is my offering to you. Welcome in. I'm truly glad you're here.

Part 1
The Overstimulated Mind

"All of humanity's problems stem from man's inability to sit quietly in a room alone."
Blaise Pascal

Chapter One
The Mental Clutter We Carry

"Your mind is like a garden. Your thoughts are the seeds. You can grow flowers, or you can grow weeds."   *- Anonymous*

If you look around you – your space, your desk, your phone screen and even within you, to navigate your thoughts, what do you find?

Notifications? To-do lists? Unfinished conversations, reminders, expectations, regrets?

Truthfully, most of us are carrying much more than we realize. Not just physically, but mentally and emotionally. And just like a cluttered room makes it hard to think clearly, a cluttered mind makes it almost impossible to be present, peaceful, or purposeful.

Welcome to that inner chaos we rarely name.

Understanding the Clutter

I see a clutter as an extreme form of disorganization; one that involves too may elements; a pile up that eventually weighs down on the subject until it becomes extremely difficult to separate on thing from the other. According to VeryWellMind,

"The word clutter refers to items that are strewn about in a disorganized fashion. In general, clutter is a collection of items that people accumulate in their homes and don't necessarily use, but hold on to anyway."

In the most subtle ways, clutters can arise from any aspect of our lives and obstruct our sense of purpose until we are all tangled up in the mess. Clutters are anything that basically stops and obstructs you from living the life you want to live and pursuing the goals that make you happy. In the presence of a clutter, you are so overwhelmed that you do not get to see through anything else and all that matters is the drowning mess.

The factor that makes a clutter different from just any distraction is its accumulation effect. The clutter does not comprise of just one thing, but a group of related – or sometimes, unrelated – entities that mix up together in areas where they do not belong. While these terms may seem relatable only in physical terms, clutters can be identified in several other spheres of life.

Different Types of Clutters

Clutters take several forms; the most relatable being physical clutters. Just think of the typical stuffs. The stuffed-up storage block of the home. The garages that can't accommodate a vehicle. The wardrobes and cupboards that can't even get shut. All these are physical clutters everywhere around us. In earlier times, I feel people tended to leave more unmaterialistic lives and were basically cool with the simple items they had. More like a simplistic type of living.

In present times, it seems like there's been a global shift and people see the need to acquire more properties with the more income they receive. While you can truly acquire as much as you wish, the element of space is vital and in no time, without proper consideration of the ratio of space to items present around you, you're bound to be jumbled up in physical clutters.

One of the most inescapable forms of clutters is the mental clutter. Trust me, you could have your space all sparky and spacious but you still can't think straight! A lot of people have been in a situation of **mental clutter** one way or the other at a moment of their lives. I've had to battle it every time. Mental clutter is the product of consistent overthinking, over-planning, over-worrying and pondering over uncertainties of life. When our minds are always flooded with the events of the past, the tension of scaling through the present and the anxiety of confronting the future, we tend to suffer mental clutter since these three tedious arms of time have become jumbled up.

Many people with complex schedules, extremely busy days and lots of plans to organize often suffer mental clutters. In a bid to juggle through everything all at once, the brain becomes weary from all the hassles and the mind suffers.

Another form of clutter closely related to the mental clutter is the **emotional clutter**. This type of weight comes from beliefs or ideals that mess up our moods and weigh us down emotionally. If you find yourself regularly getting disappointed or upset, you may be experiencing emotional clutters. Most times, these boil down to the accumulated guilt and grudges we bear in our minds, coupled with thoughts of negativity that gives us a pessimistic view of life. It gives no room for joy or freedom in our inner spirits.

Though these are the main types of clutters there are, there are also forms of **digital clutter** and **spiritual clutter**. Digital clutters are the product of our current digital age. I can imagine that those from early days, before the advent of the several clogging gadgets we use today, never had to worry about this. So, though technology comes with its many benefits, it has also come with its headaches like those glaring twenty thousand mails in your mailbox or the hundreds of unnamed files on your system that will always throw you into a hunt. These are some of the forms that digital clutter takes. Spiritual clutter and emotional clutter are very similar but with subtle differences. Spiritual clutter doesn't particularly affect your emotions but it impedes your inner being from experiencing its full potential. It hinders spiritual exploration with things that hinder the spirit like unforgiveness, guilt, shame and others.

All types of clutters come together to affect one core particularly – the mind.

The Invisible Load

There's a term psychologists use: **cognitive load**. I call it "the invisible load." It refers to the amount of mental effort being used in our working memory at any given time (Sweller, 1988). Think of it as the number of tabs open in your brain.

Now imagine that on top of your cognitive load, you also carry what sociologists call mental load. This is the invisible, ongoing work of anticipating, remembering, organizing, and planning (Daminger, 2019). This often shows up in home life, relationships, and caregiving, especially for women. It's the quiet, relentless thinking that runs underneath everything you do. As they say, "the brain never sleeps, not even when you are asleep."

Layered on top of all that? Digital clutter. Social comparison. Constant stimulation. And, of course, the noise of self-doubt, imposter syndrome, or anxiety humming in the background like a faulty refrigerator.

No, truly, there's a lot to take care of.

How the Clutters Come About

When we think about clutter, you may call it laziness or a lack of effort. The truth is that there are deeper psychological factors at play that can make tidying up feel like a challenge. I believe people hold on to their clutters due to the following reasons:

1. Feeling Overwhelmed: For many, the task of clearing things out feels too daunting. The sheer volume of items to sort through can seem intimidates them, resulting in mental and physical fatigue before they even get to anything! As a result, it can feel easier to maintain the status quo rather than face what's right in front of you.

2. Sentimental Attachments: Some bonds are rather broken, honestly. Many people hold on to items that hold significant emotional value. For example, clothes that no longer fit may be kept in the hopes of losing weight, or souvenirs from past vacations may be cherished in anticipation of future adventures. We all want to hold back that material that speaks to our memory. However, clinging to these reminders doesn't necessarily move you closer to realizing

13

those aspirations.

3. Emotional Connections to Possessions: We often retain items from our childhood or belongings that remind us of loved ones, especially if they've passed away. Letting go of these cherished objects can feel like severing connections to those memories, making it difficult to part with them.

4. Fear of Regret: The fear of regret plays a big role in people's reluctance to letting go. Many struggles with the guilt that accompanies discarding items, especially those that hold sentimental value. It's like an outcrop of the third point I made earlier; a subtle additional issue to face. Perhaps, you've thrown out some of the items and now you can't sleep properly without having it around you. That's not all; many face the anxiety of potentially needing an item in the future can lead to a habit of hanging onto things "just in case."

5. Comfort in Possessions: Our belongings often provide a sense of comfort and stability, even if they are not actively used. This emotional security can make it hard to let go, as those items create a familiar environment that feels safer than the unknown of a freer space.

6. Neurodivergent Challenges: For some individuals, particularly those with conditions like ADHD, staying organized can be particularly challenging. This can lead to a gradual accumulation of clutter, as the cognitive demands of sorting and organizing may feel overwhelming.

Hoarding Doesn't Only Happen in Commerce

Hoarding also takes place within our personal lives. My years learning my ways around the concept of clutter made me realize there is a medical term to define the inability to let go of material bonds. It's called hoarding.

Don't get it mixed up. A person who has clutter in his or her home isn't necessarily hoarding. Having clutter and having hoarding disorder are different. Still, you should look out for the signs of hoarding in yourself or those around you.

Firstly, hoarders often have cluttered areas in their homes that may prevent them from using spaces for their intended purposes, such as sleeping, cooking, or bathing. And they literally don't mind. Individuals with hoarding disorder frequently do not recognize their living conditions as problematic, which can complicate the process of seeking help.

Also, the clutter in this case can obstruct daily activities, leading to unsanitary living conditions where basic hygiene may not be maintained. Still, these hoarding behaviours persist regardless of the individual's living situation, indicating a deeper psychological challenge.

You also find signs of emotional distress among hoarders. There is often significant anxiety surrounding the thought of discarding items, contributing to a cycle of accumulation. That's plus the unsanitary conditions like accumulating food waste and trash that can lead to serious health risks, further exacerbating the living conditions and emotional states of those affected.

Understanding the Causes

Nothing in particular – at least, not one medically recognized. However, while the exact causes of hoarding disorder are not fully understood, several factors are believed to contribute such as personality traits. Traits such as indecisiveness can lead to the difficulty in making choices about what to keep or discard.

One's family history can also play a role in hoarding disorder. A background of hoarding behavior in family members may influence an individual's propensity to accumulate excessive belongings. Stressful life events have also been considered a factor to this behaviour. Significant losses (like the death of a loved one) or traumatic experiences (such as losing possessions in a disaster) can trigger or worsen hoarding behaviours. You should also understand that hoarding disorder often coexists with other mental health conditions, such as OCD and ADHD, which can complicate treatment. A study found that about 28% to 32% of those with ADHD experienced clinically significant hoarding. It was mostly recorded in those who had inattentive-type ADHD.

Quick One!

For individuals struggling with hoarding disorder, seeking help is crucial so we can just get straight into it. It's essential for them to find a supportive environment that promotes open dialogue without judgment. Here are some quick treatment options:

• Cognitive Behavioural Therapy (CBT): This therapeutic approach can help individuals change their thinking patterns about possessions and reduce anxiety related to discarding items.
• Support Groups: Connecting with others who face similar challenges can provide emotional support and practical strategies for managing hoarding behaviours.
• Professional Organizers: Specialized organizers trained to work with individuals with hoarding tendencies can assist in creating a more functional living space.

Pro-Tip: If you or someone you know exhibits signs of hoarding disorder, it's vital to approach the situation with empathy and understanding, recognizing that change is possible and support is available. That's said, let's get back on track!

You're Not Lazy; You're Overloaded

Before proceeding, let's rewrite a harmful narrative right now. You're not "bad at focusing." You're not "weak" because you feel anxious or distracted.

You're not lazy because you can't keep up.

You are simply overstimulated. Overloaded. Overwhelmed by a world that profits off your attention but rarely helps you protect it.

Author Johann Hari, in his book Stolen Focus, writes:

"We are now living in a serious attention crisis - and it's not just a personal failure, it's a systemic one" (Hari, 2022).

We weren't built for this level of input. Our minds need rest, a touch of rhythm, and constant recovery but we've been running a marathon without water breaks.

Tool: The Noise Audit

Let's carry out a little assignment. We'd be taking only 10 minutes. Grab a journal. Get honest. No editing. No judgment. We're about to access just how much clutter you may have accumulated.

1. What's been occupying my mind lately?
List everything - big or small. Tasks, worries, unfinished conversations, people, decisions.

2. What do I feel I'm constantly "behind" on?
Where do you feel pressure, guilt, or urgency?

3. What thoughts repeat daily that aren't helpful?
Notice inner scripts: "I should have..." "I'll never..." "What if..."

4. What can I release or postpone - genuinely?
Not everything is urgent. Circle what you can let go of, even temporarily.

5. What do I want more of in my mental space?
Peace? Curiosity? Joy? Inspiration? Clarity?
This simple act of naming the noise gives you back power. It's the first quiet revolution against overwhelm. There's more to come.

Conclusion

"You don't need to silence the world to find peace. You just need to stop giving everything access to your inner life."

In the next chapter, we'll explore how our devices and the tech habits we've normalized, are training our brains to crave distraction and avoid stillness. But for now, breathe.
You've already started the work.

Chapter Two
Tech Addiction Is Stealing Your Attention

Research found that nearly 95% of teens in the United States have access to smartphones, and many are concerned about overusing them.

-Pew Research Center

95%? Wow!

Welcome to the 21st century; the age of infinite scrolling. We are living in the most connected time in human history and yet, many of us feel deeply disconnected. This is one of the greatest ironies of human history, at least to me.

We are disconnected from ourselves. Disconnected from purpose. Disconnected from the still, quiet corners of life where we find true clarity. I recall there was once a time when you could walk down the street and interact with other humans – ordinary people living ordinary lives.

Now?

We scroll. We scroll in line, while eating, during conversations, and often without even realizing it. It's called infinite scroll for a reason. There's no end. No natural stopping point. No pause. And that's precisely the point. This chapter digs into the aspect of digital clutter with tech addiction being at its nucleus.

From the Village Square to the Digital Feed

Let's rewind a few generations. Life wasn't easier, yeah. I mean, you couldn't exactly just speak to anyone from the comfort of your home or press a couple of keys and have hours of tasks finished in minutes. It was simpler though. I remember routines and natural pauses in the day that invited reflection. Some of these moments were walking to school, writing letters (cheesy, but very much heartfelt), or sitting by a fire after sundown.

The community that many elderly individuals today once experienced was face-to-face. Things like news came in measured doses. And when you were alone, you were just... alone. It did not necessarily mean you were lonely or disconnected. Here's how I call it – you were present with yourself.

Compare that to today, where self-presence feels like a lost art. The "village square" has been replaced by comment sections. I mean, what is the need to express one another face-to-face when we could just type a couple comments right? Family conversations have been replaced by individual screens glowing in their faces alone. Skip those TV commercials where a happy family sit cuddled together in front of a screen. Our realistic world knows that's not just true. Even moments of grief, celebration, or crisis are filtered through a lens of "What should I post about this?"

Nope!

We have never had so much access to information and yet so little space to digest it. In his book Amusing Ourselves to Death, Neil Postman predicted this cultural shift back in 1985. He warned that our appetite for constant entertainment would dull our critical thinking and reduce everything to spectacle. He writes:

"What Orwell feared were those who would ban books. What Huxley feared was that there would be no reason to ban a book, for there would be no one who wanted to read one." (Postman, 1985). It's not that we don't have time to think anymore.
It's that our time is being slowly consumed by distraction masquerading as connection.

The Illusion of Productivity

Perhaps the most dangerous part of this digital noise is that it feels like we're doing something valuable. Social media already gives you that "sense" of satisfaction that tells your mind, "Yeah, I'm making progress!"

You open your phone to check the weather report and suddenly you're ten videos deep into a feed. Seriously? You respond to a message and thirty minutes vanish inside a rabbit hole of content. For real? You read an article but forget what it said by the time you switch apps.

It's not laziness. It's design.

Apps are built to hold your gaze. They prey on your attention, harness your impulses, and reward your brain for staying longer than you intended. They offer the illusion of productivity, learning, and engagement while slowly eroding your capacity for deep focus.

And here's what's most important: this isn't happening by accident.

Our attention is being fractured into a thousand tiny pieces. Author and researcher Cal Newport calls this phenomenon "attention residue" - when fragments of our focus linger on the last thing we saw, making it harder to transition into deep or meaningful thought (Newport, 2016). That explains why we struggle to pray, meditate, write, think, or even finish a full sentence in our journal without wanting to check something "really quick."

The Science Behind Screen Addiction

"The chains of habit are too weak to be felt until they are too strong to be broken."   - Samuel Johnson

It's easy to believe that we're just "bad at focusing." That we need more discipline. More self-control. A better alarm app. But science tells us otherwise. In reality, the designers of the so-called social media platforms we use are psychologists; they understand the workings of the brain. How else can the operation of these platforms be profitable for them if they do not have the huge number of people that keep using these applications? That's why they designed them diligently in line with the rules of neuroscience.

Dopamine: The Brain's Reward Currency

Let's start with the brain chemical that shows up in nearly every conversation about addiction: **dopamine**. Contrary to popular belief, dopamine isn't the chemical of pleasure. It's the chemical of anticipation. It's what spikes when you expect a reward, not necessarily when you get it.

Each time you hear a notification ding, get a like on a photo, or stumble across something mildly interesting online, your brain gives you a little dopamine hit – that nudge of curiosity that says, "Ooh, let's see what's next." So, it's no accident. The infinite scroll, autoplay, random rewards (likes, comments, new content) all mimic the psychological mechanisms of gambling.

According to Dr. Anna Lembke, professor of psychiatry at Stanford University and author of *Dopamine Nation*,

"We are now all vulnerable to compulsive overconsumption - not just of drugs and alcohol but of digital content that is immediately available, incredibly potent, and highly rewarding" (Lembke, 2021, p. 10).

The more you use your device in short bursts – scroll, swipe, click, repeat – the more your brain learns to seek stimulation, not satisfaction. It's like standing in front of a vending machine that never runs out, even if you're full.

Neuroplasticity and the Rewiring of Focus

Still being brain scientists, let's explore another term. This part might pinch a little. Here's the double-edged sword: your brain is incredibly adaptable. It can literally rewire itself based on what you repeatedly do. This is called **neuroplasticity**. Neuroplasticity, in simple terms, is the brain's ability to form new neural pathways. So, what happens when you check your phone 96 times a day (the current global average, according to Asurion, 2019)? Or jump from app to app 7–10 times per hour? You start training your brain to crave fragmentation. Your attention span shrinks. You become less comfortable with stillness, and more comfortable with noise.

In his book *The Shallows, Nicholas Carr writes:*

"The more we use the Web, the more we train our brain to be distracted - to process information quickly and superficially" (Carr, 2010, p. 120).

Your focus becomes shallow. Your thinking becomes scattered. And over time, deep work such as writing, reflecting, reading, praying, and thinking, feels too slow for your turbo-trained mind.

Ay, are you having issues taking note as you read? Take a pause. Do you see it now? Now, let's move on.

Attention Residue and Mental Fatigue

When we jump between tasks, we don't reset cleanly. We carry little fragments of the previous task with us such as lingering questions, half-formed ideas, leftover emotions.

This is called **attention residue**, a term coined by researcher Sophie Leroy.
And it's why multitasking often feels productive but is actually draining your brain's resources and slowing your thinking (Leroy, 2009).
So, when you check your messages in the middle of a focused task, a part of your brain doesn't return with you right away. It lags behind. Over time, that lag builds up, leading to what we now call **digital fatigue** which translates into a sense of dullness, restlessness, or emotional fog caused not by exhaustion, but overstimulation.

It's no wonder that even on days when you don't do "much," you feel *mentally exhausted* by 4 p.m. Trust me, I had to battle with this for so long!

Why This Isn't Just About "Too Much Screen Time"

All these isn't just about time. It's about the quality of engagement. You could spend hours watching a movie with someone you love and feel enriched. But spend 15 minutes jumping between 5 apps and you feel wired, anxious, and strangely empty.

Why? Because passive, fractured stimulation isn't the same as meaningful engagement. Dr. Gloria Mark, an expert in digital distraction, found in her research that the average knowledge worker switches task every three minutes, and that it can take over 23 minutes to get fully back into focus (Mark et al., 2008). That's 23 minutes of mental residue from a simple distraction like a text or tweet. In her recent book *Attention Span*, Mark goes on to say:

"We are operating in a state of perpetual cognitive whiplash."

We are constantly context switching, constantly self-interrupting, constantly checking, reacting, clicking, updating. And this fragmented state becomes our new normal until we forget what it felt like to be *fully present* in anything.

The Cost of Constant Connection

At first, being constantly connected feels empowering. It's like you've got the world at your fingertips! To be honest, the global connectivity of this century has been the landmark of several inventions and the expansion of knowledge. You're reachable. You're informed. You're engaged. But over time, something shifts.

You stop feeling connected to yourself. Because that's the paradox: The more connected we become digitally, the more disconnected we risk becoming emotionally, relationally, and even spiritually.

"We turn to our phones instead of each other, and in the process, we sacrifice conversation for mere connection. But connection without conversation doesn't nurture us - it leaves us lonely." (Turkle, 2015, p. 3)

Relationships: Together, But Alone

Let's do a little dive in into our relationships. Have you ever seen a couple at dinner, both scrolling? Or sat in a room with friends, each absorbed in their own screen?

Have you ever been mid-conversation and watched someone glance down "just for a second" - and the moment was lost? We don't mean to disconnect from each other.

But we've allowed our devices to become third parties in our relationships.

This has real consequences. According to a 2021 Pew Research study, nearly 4 in 10 adults say they feel less connected to others now than before the rise of social media, despite interacting online more frequently (Pew Research Center, 2021).

Dr. Jean Twenge, a psychologist known for studying generational shifts, found that adolescents who spent more than 3 hours a day on devices were significantly more likely to report symptoms of anxiety, depression, and loneliness (Twenge & Campbell, 2018).

Self-Worth in the Age of Comparison

Let's talk about the emotional tax we pay to "keep up."

You didn't used to know what your old classmate's living room looked like, or what your ex is doing for brunch, or how someone else's child is developing compared to yours.

But now you do.

And whether we admit it or not, comparison is unavoidable in digital spaces. Not because we're jealous or shallow but because our brains are wired to **benchmark**. To measure where we are by observing others.

Social media intensifies that instinct, but it only shows what I would call the highlight reel. This is the filtered, edited, carefully selected moments of people's lives. We compare our behind-the-scenes mess to their polished, front-stage moments. And unsurprisingly, we come up short. This quiet comparison culture has been linked to increasing levels of:

- Low self-esteem

- Impostor syndrome

- Perfectionism

- FOMO (fear of missing out)

And it's not limited to teens. Adults are equally susceptible. As researcher Brené Brown puts it:

"Stay in your lane. Comparison kills creativity and joy."

And beyond creativity and joy? It also steals rest. Because you're constantly assessing: Am I doing enough? Am I falling behind? Am I missing out?

Overwiring the Nervous System

Our minds aren't the only things affected by this constant connection.

Our bodies feel it too. Endless alerts, notifications, and dopamine loops keep us in a low-grade fight-or-flight mode. Our nervous systems are revved up constantly, even when we're not in danger. You may notice symptoms like:

- Irritability or restlessness

- Difficulty falling asleep

- Chronic fatigue

- Increased anxiety or brain fog

- A nagging sense that you should be doing something else

According to Dr. Stephen Porges' *Polyvagal Theory*, our bodies are wired to feel safe when we experience slowness, eye contact, and co-regulation with others. But constant digital input bypasses those cues and keeps us in a heightened state of alert (Porges, 2011). In simpler terms: Your phone may be hijacking your body's sense of safety!

Big Tech and the Attention Economy

"If you're not paying for the product, you are the product."
- *Common adage about the internet economy*

Let's be honest: most of us didn't sign up for a life of distraction.

We didn't choose to be chronically overstimulated nor did we consciously decide to train our brains to crave swipes and scrolls. And yet, here we are, living in an age where quiet feels uncomfortable, and full presence feels foreign. But to truly understand how we got here, we have to ask a bigger question:

Who profits when your attention is fractured? Big Tech.

The Marketplace of Attention

In the past, the economy revolved around goods and labour. Today, we live in what many experts call the attention economy which is a marketplace where your focus is the most valuable commodity. Every notification, vibration, autoplay video, or algorithmic suggestion is designed with one purpose in mind: To keep you on the platform.

Why? Because your time = their money.

The longer you stay, the more ads you see. The more ads you see, the more money they make. In his groundbreaking book *Ten Arguments for Deleting Your Social Media Accounts Right Now*, Jaron Lanier (a founding figure in virtual reality and former Silicon Valley insider) calls this the "behavioural modification market."

He writes:

"It's not just that your attention is being bought and sold; it's that you are being subtly changed by what you see, in order to keep you seeing more of it." (Lanier, 2018, p. 32)

Surveillance Capitalism: The Business of You

Harvard professor Shoshana Zuboff coined the term "surveillance capitalism" to describe the practice of collecting massive amounts of personal data, not just what you click, but how long you pause, what you scroll past, what emojis you use, what time of day you're active, and even your facial expressions on video.

These companies don't just store this data but they sell it as well. It's used to predict your behavior, customize your feed, and nudge your emotions, all in the service of keeping you engaged.

Zuboff explains:

"The goal of surveillance capitalism is to automate us. To shape our behavior in the direction of maximum profit, without our awareness and without our consent." (The Age of Surveillance Capitalism, 2019) That means your digital environment is not neutral. It is rather engineered. Understand that your feeds, your timelines, your recommendations and everything else are not random. They're curated for addiction, for polarization and for profit.

In 2020, The Social Dilemma documentary pulled back the curtain on how platforms like Facebook, Instagram, TikTok, and YouTube use AI to manipulate engagement. Former Google design ethicist Tristan Harris revealed that these companies hire neuroscientists, behavioural psychologists, and persuasive designers to maximize "time on platform."

"It's not a fair fight between our brains and the technology. We have

palaeolithic emotions, medieval institutions, and god-like technology."
In all, we're all up against a system designed to win.

That's one terrible fight.

Tool: The Digital Boundaries Blueprint

It's about time you crafted a screen-use strategy that honours your attention, protects your peace, and reconnects you with what matters.

"Boundaries are the distance at which I can love you and me simultaneously."
- Prentis Hemphill

We've talked about how technology is hijacking your attention. Now, it's time to reclaim it and we won't be going through some drastic digital cleanses or unrealistic detoxes. I want us to do something more sustainable. I call it "intentional boundaries."

You don't need to toss your phone in a lake. Oh no! You just need to decide what gets access to your inner life and, of course, when! So grab your journal or Notes app. Let's walk through a five-part process to craft your own Digital Boundaries Blueprint.

Step 1: Audit Your Attention

Before you create new boundaries, you need to know where your attention is going now. For the next 24 hours:

- Track how often you check your phone or scroll aimlessly.

- List your top 3 most-used apps (check Screen Time or Digital Wellbeing settings).

- Notice: When do you reach for your phone the most: boredom? anxiety? avoidance?

Reflection prompts:

- What am I really looking for when I check my phone?

- What part of my life or mind am I trying to escape?

- What do I feel after I scroll: energized or drained?

Step 2: Define Your Digital Values

Now ask yourself: What do I want my relationship with tech to look like?

Pick 2–3 core values to guide your screen use. Some examples:

- Presence: "I want to be fully available in conversations."

- Rest: "I want my evenings to feel restorative, not rushed."

- Focus: "I want to reclaim deep work and creative time."

- Joy: "I want to use tech for connection, not comparison."

Write them down. These will be your compass. When your usage habits begin to drift, your values will bring you home.

Step 3: Set Micro-Boundaries

Here's where it gets practical. For each of the digital "leaks" in your life, set tiny, sustainable boundaries. The brain loves small tasks. It will draw you closer to achievement.

Examples:

• App Limits: "I will use Instagram only between 6–7 p.m."

• No-Phone Zones: "No phones at the dinner table or in bed."

• Notification Control: "I will turn off all non-essential app notifications."

• Focused Mornings: "No screens for the first 30 minutes of my day."

• One Screen Rule: "No scrolling while watching shows: one device at a time."

Pro tip: Start small. Don't try to overhaul everything overnight. Pick one or two micro-boundaries this week and test how it feels.

Step 4: Replace, Don't Just Remove

A boundary without a nourishing alternative becomes a void. Read that again! So ask yourself: What am I unplugging FOR?

Replace screen time with analogue joy:

• Morning scroll: journaling or stretching

• Doomscrolling at night: reading fiction or sipping tea in silence

• Habitual Instagram breaks: stepping outside for 5 minutes

• Group chats: a phone call with one real friend

Step 5: Communicate Your Boundaries

Let people know what you're doing and why especially family, friends, or coworkers who are used to immediate responses. Example messages:

•   "I'm stepping back from my phone after 8 p.m. to protect my sleep. You can always reach me before then."

•   "I won't be checking emails on weekends to recharge. Thanks for understanding!"

Conclusion

"My attention is mine to protect. My peace is worth preserving. I am allowed to disconnect to reconnect."

If you're feeling refreshed, we're only getting started. In the next chapter, we'll be exploring the cost of these mental clutters and the signs that you are weighed down by the overload.

Chapter Three
Anxiety, Burnout, and the Modern Mind

You know that feeling when everything should be fine? Big emphasis on "should." I mean, you've ticked off the to-do list. Everyone around you says you're doing great. You post the right things, respond to your texts, show up for work or school, handle your responsibilities. You even smile when someone asks, "How are you?"

But underneath, something feels... off. It feels like your chest is carrying a tightness it doesn't know how to name. It feels like you're running on fumes, but from what, exactly? You can't even tell.

This chapter is about that feeling. I call it the quiet hum of modern anxiety; the fatigue that doesn't go away with sleep; the ache of living in a world that praises busyness but forgets to check if you're okay. Let's name it together.

An Invisible Exhaustion

On a Tuesday morning in suburban Maryland, 34-year-old Nicole sat in her SUV in the Target parking lot with her forehead pressed against the steering wheel. She wasn't crying. She wasn't panicking. She wasn't even sure what she was doing.

She had just dropped the kids off at school. She had groceries to grab, emails to answer, and a Zoom call in an hour. But instead, there she was... frozen in a strip mall parking lot, unable to move.

To anyone watching, Nicole was holding it all together. Her LinkedIn page still sparkled with career wins. Her Instagram was full of sweet family moments and perfectly lit coffee cups. Her neighbours admired how "on top of things" she always seemed.

But lately, she couldn't concentrate. Her sleep was shallow. Her thoughts kept looping: Did I respond to that email? Did I sign the permission slip? Did I forget something again?

Somewhere between school drop-off and the cereal aisle, Nicole's body whispered what her brain had been ignoring: "I'm done."

This is just one basic story, taking root from the true conversation I once had with a young woman I'd rather keep anonymous. However, from this excerpt, there's something very tentative to draw on.

You don't have to be a mother to relate to Nicole. Maybe you're a student juggling classes, side hustles, and the silent pressure to have your life figured out by twenty-three. Maybe you're a caregiver for a parent, a manager in an always-on company, or simply a person trying to hold it together in a world that never stops spinning.

Invisible exhaustion doesn't always look dramatic. Sometimes, it looks like forgetting what you just walked into a room for. Sometimes, it looks like laughing at a joke but not really feeling it. Other times, it looks like doing everything right but feeling nothing at all.

There's a name for what you're feeling. It's called functional anxiety. This is a quiet, high-functioning kind of unrest that hides in plain sight. It thrives in people who are reliable, over-responsible, and constantly moving. It sounds like:

- "I'm fine. Just tired."
- "I don't know why I feel this way. Everything's going okay."
- "I should be grateful. Other people have it worse."

But functional doesn't mean healthy. Doing the thing doesn't mean you're okay doing the thing. And pushing through isn't the same as healing.

Let's pause here and get honest.

When was the last time you felt present? Not just there physically but emotionally at home in your body, not multitasking in your head?

When was the last time you woke up and didn't feel behind?

When was the last time you didn't immediately reach for your phone, just to fill the silence? That's the invisible exhaustion. It creeps in when we stop checking in with ourselves and start surviving by muscle memory. It thrives when we're too busy to notice our own unravelling.

The Anatomy of Burnout

I won't call "burnout" the mere feeling of being tired. More like being burnt-out!

It's a full-body, full-soul depletion that doesn't go away with a nap or a weekend off.

Defined by the World Health Organization (2019) as an *occupational phenomenon,* burnout results from chronic workplace stress that has not been successfully managed. But in real life, burnout isn't limited to your job title. It affects students, parents, freelancers, caretakers, and yes – even people who love what they do.

At its core, burnout is what happens when we push past our inner red flags too long. It's your body saying *"I'm not okay"* in every way it knows how, either through fatigue, or through disinterest, restlessness, brain fog, aches, apathy, name it.

Researchers Maslach and Leiter (1997), who pioneered one of the most widely accepted models for understanding burnout, broke it down into three major dimensions. Let's look at them closely.

Emotional Exhaustion

This is usually where it starts. It is the steady depletion of your emotional energy. It's the feeling of running on empty. It is like you've got nothing left to give, but life keeps asking. You wake up tired, go through your day tired, and crawl into bed with a mind that won't stop racing.

It's different from regular fatigue. This kind of tired lives deep in your chest. It dulls your joy. It makes small tasks feel heavy and normal interactions feel draining.

Nicole, from the earlier story, felt it in her bones such that speaking wasn't even feasible. And maybe you have too – when answering one more email makes you want to scream, or when showing up to that Zoom meeting feels like a betrayal to your nervous system.

It's not because you're not capable but more like your emotional well has been running dry for too long.

Depersonalization / Cynicism

When emotional exhaustion is left unchecked, it often gives way to detachment.

You stop caring and it's not because you're cruel or cold but because it's the only way your system knows how to survive. You put walls up. You go numb. You show up physically, but emotionally you've clocked out.

This is called depersonalization, a defence mechanism that creates emotional distance from the people or responsibilities that used to matter to you.

You might find yourself snapping at coworkers or loved ones. You might become sarcastic, cynical, or apathetic. You might say things like:

- "It doesn't matter anyway."
- "Nobody cares, so why should I?"
- "I just don't have it in me anymore."

You become someone you barely recognize but don't have the energy to change.

And here's the kicker: the more you disconnect, the more isolated and guilty you feel. It becomes a cruel loop.

Reduced Personal Accomplishment

This final dimension is the quiet killer of motivation. You start to doubt yourself. Even if you're still producing or showing up, it doesn't feel like enough. You question your worth, your competence, your progress. You might find yourself thinking:

- "I should be doing more."

- "I'm falling behind."
- "What's the point?"

Imposter syndrome flares and satisfaction fades. You stop celebrating your wins, or worse, you stop believing they matter at all.

And ironically, guess the people most vulnerable to this stage? They are the high-achievers, the helpers, the perfectionists. The people who once found meaning in their work are the ones who feel its loss most deeply when burnout strikes.

These three dimensions revolve around five stages.

The Five Stages of Burnout

Burnout doesn't happen overnight. It's not like flipping a switch. Let me say it is more like a slow dimming of the lights. You begin bright-eyed and full of energy and if the stress isn't managed, or if the pace becomes unsustainable and the pressure unchecked, that initial spark fades. This will all take place so subtly and slowly; you'll be all good and okay, and then – boom! You find yourself barely lit at all.

Here's what that dimming often looks like:

The Honeymoon Phase

You're starting a new job or launching a business or diving into a passion project. Maybe you're even stepping into a caregiving role for a loved one with a full heart.

At this stage, you're energized and optimistic. You're driven. You feel purposeful. Maybe a little invincible. You say yes to everything. You work late. You skip lunch. You push your limits because, at this point, it feels good.

Stress exists, but it's manageable. You may even enjoy the pressure; it feels like growth. I've been there and I've once loved that bustling atmosphere. For me, it meant success.

However, the danger of the Honeymoon Phase is that we ignore the warning signs. We tell ourselves we'll rest "after this season," not realizing the season is becoming our lifestyle.

Onset of Stress

This is when the cracks begin to show.

You start waking up tired. Your patience thins. Tasks that once excited you now feel like obligations. You might find yourself drinking more coffee, zoning out during conversations, or forgetting little things like where you placed your keys, what day that meeting was, why you walked into the room.

You're still functioning, but the stress is no longer just background noise. It's now creeping into your habits, your health, your moods.

You may begin to notice things like sleep disturbances, muscle tension or headaches, avoidance tendencies, or more commonly, a general sense of overwhelm

This is your body's way of whispering, "*Hey... this is too much.*"

Chronic Stress

The whisper has turned into a murmur that never stops. At this stage, stress is no longer situational but systemic. It's not one bad week. It's your new normal.

You may experience signs like persistent fatigue, difficulty concentrating, emotional irritability, increased conflict in relationships, cynicism or detachment

This is the point where many people begin to withdraw emotionally. You start to feel numb. Tasks blur together. Days pass without you really feeling them.

You keep pushing, because that's what you've always done but inside, you know something's wrong.

Burnout Phase

This is full-blown burnout. All the warning signs have crescendo into a loud, crashing wave. You feel emotionally, mentally, and physically exhausted. You may dread getting out of bed. You may cry easily or not at all, because you feel too numb to cry.

The three key symptoms from earlier (emotional exhaustion, depersonalization, and reduced accomplishment) are now deeply rooted.

In this phase, many people begin to feel ashamed or lost. They question their worth. They may consider quitting their job, ghosting responsibilities, or isolating from loved ones. They often feel like they're failing even if no one else sees it that way.

This is when many people finally reach out for help or collapse from not doing so sooner. Because, God help us, there's a fifth stage!

Habitual Burnout

This is the most dangerous stage not because it's explosive, but because it's quiet and lethal. Habitual burnout is what happens when burnout becomes a way of life. You adapt to the exhaustion. You normalize the brain fog. You start believing this is just who you are now: distracted, anxious, joyless.

Your nervous system becomes locked in survival mode. You may experience long-term consequences:
- Depression or chronic anxiety
- Frequent illness or physical pain
- Digestive issues, inflammation, or sleep disorders
- Disconnection from your goals, identity, or sense of self

This is where burnout sinks its roots. And unless intentionally interrupted, it can affect every domain of your life: work, relationships, creativity, health, joy.

Forever...

Pro-Tip: Every stage is reversible though.

Even if you're in the later stages, your body and mind are designed for healing. You may not bounce back overnight, but with awareness, support, and small shifts in how you treat yourself, recovery is possible.

Now let's explore one of the biggest accelerators of burnout in our modern world: the pressure to perform - constantly - for approval, productivity, or worth.

The Performance Trap

You don't even remember when it started; when doing your best slowly turned into proving your worth. At first, it was innocent. Maybe you liked gold stars. Maybe you were the helpful one. Maybe achievement gave you a sense of safety in a world that felt unpredictable.

However, somewhere along the way, effort became identity. You learned that being useful was how you stayed accepted, that being productive was how you stayed valued, that being perfect was how you stayed safe.

So you performed.

I've been in this scenario and I will liken it to the life of a celebrity figure we see on TV. From my encounter with artistic performers, sometimes referred to as thespians, they have a particular saying that, "the show must go on." This statement implied that irrespective of the internal or external forces that may hinder the performer, he was still urged to deliver flawlessly.

You showed up even when your body said rest. You smiled when your heart felt heavy. You chased promotions, poured into others, responded with "no worries!" when there definitely were worries because being okay became part of your brand.

And here's the tricky thing: it worked. You got praise. You got opportunities. You got liked. But inside, a quiet question started to echo: "Who am I if I stop?"

Performance as a Coping Strategy

In one of the sessions I had with such theatrical performer, he highlighted that sometimes, actually performing and delivering served as "temporary" relief to the burden and stress he feels. It was like a medicine that only lasted a while.

Many of us grew up equating performance with survival. Maybe your home rewarded perfection. Maybe school taught you that your GPA mattered more than your feelings. Or culture taught you to hustle, grind, and optimize every corner of your life because rest is for the lazy and boundaries are for the weak.

So you became the reliable one. The responsible one. The one people could always count on. But here's what no one told you: The performance doesn't end just because the curtain closes. If you're not careful, you start living on stage - all the time.

When Worth Gets Tied to Output

What happens when your self-worth is tied to your output?

You stop asking what brings you joy. You stop asking how you feel.

You start evaluating yourself based on numbers: followers, income, checklists, calories, grades. You become data about yourself - not in connection with yourself.

You begin performing not just for your boss or your family, but for strangers on the internet. And boy, does it ever end? Because performance always demands more.

The Loop: Do More → Be More → Feel Less

The Performance Trap is a loop that looks like this:

1. **You feel pressure to do more.**
2. **You start achieving to prove yourself.**
3. **You get praised for it.**
4. **You raise your standards even higher.**
5. **You begin to disconnect from your actual needs.**
6. **You feel even more pressure to do more.**

Stress Hormones and the Overstimulated Nervous System

Now, the tricky part about the stress is that even when you've got it all covered in the mind, you really don't escape the effect on your body. Even if your mind tries to power through the noise, your body keeps score.

What are you picturing? Let me guess: that low-grade anxiety? Or is it the shallow breaths? The tension in your neck and shoulders? The racing thoughts at 2:00 a.m.? These aren't random symptoms but your body trying to communicate what your mind is struggling to ignore. They're physiological signals; evidence that your nervous system has been living in survival mode for too long.

Let's take a moment to understand what's happening under the hood when stress becomes chronic.

Your Body's Stress Response: A Brilliant Survival System

The human body is wired to survive threats. When danger shows up, whether it's a tiger in the wild or a critical email from your boss, your brain signals a cascade of hormonal responses known as the stress response (Sapolsky, 2004).

Here's what happens:

1.   The amygdala, the brain's fear center, senses a threat.

2.   It alerts the hypothalamus, which kicks off a message to your adrenal glands.

3.   These glands then release stress hormones like adrenaline and cortisol into your bloodstream.

These hormones prepare you to either fight, flee, or freeze:

• Your heart races to pump more blood to muscles.

• Your pupils dilate to sharpen focus.

• Digestion slows down (because who needs a snack during a lion chase?).

• And your brain becomes hyper-alert.

In a real emergency, this is brilliant. It can save your life. But when this system is constantly activated by modern stressors like deadlines, social media, traffic, bills, performance anxiety, it turns toxic. Your brain and body can't tell the difference between a life-threatening event and a full inbox and when you're always in a heightened state of alert, your nervous system becomes dysregulated.

Chronic Cortisol: The Silent Agitator

One of the most well-studied hormones in stress science is cortisol commonly referred to as the "stress hormone." While helpful in short bursts, prolonged cortisol elevation can wreak havoc on your health (McEwen, 2006).

Chronic cortisol exposure has been linked to:

• Fatigue and insomnia

• Brain fog and memory issues

• Suppressed immune function

• Increased belly fat

• Hormonal imbalances

• Anxiety and mood instability

It can even shrink the hippocampus, the part of your brain responsible for memory and learning (Lupien et al., 2009). So bear in mind that long-term stress literally rewires your brain.

The Overstimulated Nervous System

The autonomic nervous system which regulates involuntary bodily functions like heart rate, digestion, and breathing has two main branches:

• The sympathetic nervous system ("fight or flight")

• The parasympathetic nervous system ("rest and digest")

In a healthy body, these systems balance each other out but in burnout, the sympathetic system becomes dominant, leaving the parasympathetic system underused and underdeveloped. You get stuck in a loop of hypervigilance. Even when nothing's objectively wrong, your body keeps acting like danger is around the corner. So next time when you feel so paranoid and always on the lookout, remember that – nope, you're not a superhero with some mystical abilities... you're stressed.

This can show up as:

- Hyperactivity or restlessness
- Panic attacks or irritability
- Difficulty relaxing or falling asleep
- Emotional numbing
- Digestive problems (because rest-and-digest is offline)

Tool: The Energy Check-In

Let's call this a daily body-mind scan to tune into your needs

"The body whispers before it screams."

- Unknown

So many of us spend our days reacting to life instead of responding to it.

We charge through emails, errands, and expectations, rarely asking ourselves one powerful question: **How am I, really?**

This is what the Energy Check-In is here to do: Let's bring you back to yourself, at least before your body has to shut down to get your attention.

You don't need a quiet mountain or a full hour. For this exercise of mine, you only need 5–10 honest, uninterrupted minutes.

Try this once a day: in the morning, during a lunch break, or just before bed.

Here are your tools: a journal (or the Notes app), your breath, and, yeah, some compassion.

Step 1: Check in With Your Body

Start with a few slow breaths. Feel your feet on the ground. Drop your shoulders. Close your eyes if it feels safe.

Then ask yourself:

- What physical sensations am I feeling right now? (Tension?

Fatigue? Lightness? Aches? Energy?)

- Where in my body do I feel most activated or most relaxed?
- Am I hungry, thirsty, rested, or overstimulated?

Step 2: Check in With Your Mind

Now tune into your mental space:

- What thoughts are on loop today?
- Am I feeling clear or scattered? Focused or fuzzy?
- What's one thing taking up the most mental space?
- What's something I can set down even temporarily?

Step 3: Check in With Your Heart

Now turn inward:

- What emotions are present? (Name them: joy, anxiety, irritation, hope, numbness.)
- Do I feel connected... or disconnected?
- What am I needing emotionally right now? (Support? Encouragement? Space? Reassurance?)

If nothing comes up, that's okay. Numbness is a feeling too and often a sign you're overwhelmed.

Step 4: Choose One Gentle Response

Based on what came up, ask:

- What's one thing I can do to support myself today?

Examples:

- Stretch for five minutes.
- Cancel a non-essential commitment.
- Listen to calming music.
- Reach out to someone I trust.
- Write something that's been stuck inside.
- Do one task mindfully.

- Do nothing - on purpose.

Don't consider this a to-do list but a to-care list and let's move one step closer to your total wellbeing.

Conclusion

You don't have to wait until you're running on fumes to pause.

I consider checking in with your body, mind, and heart a daily act of self-respect. Rest isn't a reward for finally doing enough. Let's call it a rhythm; one that helps you become enough without burning out. However, all these are only the prologue to the healing process. Now, are we set for a full detox – for a decluttering exercise?

Part II
The Decluttering Journey

"Almost everything will work again if you unplug it for a few minutes, including you."
- Anne Lamott

Chapter Four
The Art of Decluttering

It's been quite the discussion about understanding what it means to be enveloped in clutters and how the mismanagement of this situation can potentially wreck your life. The good thing, though, is that there's a positive side to this. You are actually in total control.

Yes, it's easy to feel like whatever situation you're presently in is much beyond your scope, but as we've learnt, that's basically what clutters do – they overwhelm you. This is the reason why we've extensively discussed what it means to be cluttered and stuffed in every sphere of life. Like one would say, "Know thy enemy!" It's a good thing we now know and understand what we're dealing with. Now is the moment to understand the weapon needed to put the enemy under control.

Let's get straight to it!

The Hidden Power of Letting Go

Quick story time!

I once lived in a tiny apartment tucked between two noisy roads. Just close your eyes and picture one of those places where silence was never guaranteed, and the kitchen counter doubled as a desk, therapy corner, and tea station. I was freelancing at the time, trying to meet writing deadlines while also navigating a season of personal transition that left me feeling scattered and slightly hollow.

What I didn't realize then was that my space had become a mirror of my mind.

The dining table was littered with receipts I hadn't filed, half-read books I felt guilty for not finishing, and a stack of unopened mail I told myself I'd "get to soon." My closet held clothes I hadn't worn in years but kept "just in case." My digital life wasn't any better. We're talking tabs upon tabs open in my browser, notes scattered across three different apps, a phone that buzzed more often than I breathed.

It wasn't that I was lazy. If anything, I was always doing something. But I began to notice that I was rarely *fully* present with anything. My thoughts were as cluttered as my surroundings: fragmented, anxious, unfinished.

One afternoon, I sat down at my table to write and couldn't focus. I stared at the screen, then at the chaos around me, and suddenly felt suffocated by the weight of things I had long ignored. So, I did something simple: I cleared the table. I threw away the junk mail, shelved the books without guilt, wiped the surface clean. Ten minutes later, I sat back down and exhaled, as if for the first time in weeks.

That was the moment I realized: the clutter wasn't just around me; it was inside me. My physical world was a projection of my inner turbulence. And by making space in the physical, I was learning how to make space in the emotional. What began as a quick tidying session became a much deeper shift. I started asking more intentional questions: *Why am I holding onto this? What story does this object (or belief, or habit) keep alive?* The more I cleared, the more I came back to myself.

Decluttering is a form of lightening. not only our shelves but our spirits.

To declutter is to practice discernment. It's to say, "This belongs, this doesn't." It's to reclaim authority over your time, energy, and attention. It's to step out of autopilot and into conscious curation of your environment, your habits, your thoughts. In a way, decluttering is about asking better questions: Do I need this or have I just gotten used to it? Does this belief, pattern, or possession reflect who I am now? What would I feel if I released this: relief, fear, guilt, freedom?

These questions are what I term "questions of alignment." Their answers pull you back to a beginning where clarity ruled. They're about recognizing that every single thing you keep, whether physical or psychological, takes up space. And you only have so much.

When we make space, we make room for life to breathe again. We gain clarity not just from what we remove, but from the quiet that remains after the noise is gone. And in that quiet, we begin to remember who we are underneath the clutter.

The Pros of Decluttering – A Checklist for Company

I won't take you through a series of the traumatizing negativity of clutter without giving you the positive gains of embarking on your decluttering journey. As a matter of fact, you're meant to experience seven out of the eleven benefits given below. So, before each benefit is a checkbox which you're to tick out once you've experienced it in your decluttering journey. So bookmark this page, because you'll be coming all the way back to access just how far you've come when we begin to clean that mess up!

First and foremost, decluttering promotes your **overall well-being**, providing a fertile ground for creativity and inspiration to flourish. A tidy space fosters emotional health by alleviating feelings of overwhelm and reducing anxiety. By decluttering, you're creating a calming retreat that enhances focus and productivity. On top of that, a neat environment can significantly improve sleep quality, allowing for much-needed rest and rejuvenation.

Transitioning to a cleaner environment **enhances safety** by clearing tripping hazards and ensuring a smoother evacuation during emergencies. A decluttered space opens new avenues for exercise and meditation, supports a robust immune system by reducing germs, and simplifies cleaning tasks, making them less of a chore. Plus, by encouraging responsible disposal methods, decluttering aligns with sustainable practices, reducing waste and supporting ethical consumption, ultimately contributing to a healthier planet.

Moreover, decluttering can yield substantial **financial benefits**. I know, you're already wondering, "I can really get richer by clearing out stuffs?" Well, yeah... in a way. By minimizing possessions, you reduce maintenance and repair costs while enhancing your home's energy efficiency, leading to lower utility bills. The process also allows you to discover valuable items to sell, providing an unexpected boost to your finances. Furthermore, an organized space helps prevent unnecessary purchases, encouraging a more mindful approach to spending.

One of the best things I enjoyed from decluttering is having a **peaceful and inviting living space.** I could more freely welcome people to my home at any time. It reflects your values and lifestyle, fostering a home that radiates positive energy and readiness for any emergencies. By decluttering, each corner of your home can become a representation of intentional living.

On a personal level, decluttering encourages **personal growth and self-discovery**. It allows individuals to rekindle forgotten interests and passions while fostering awareness and mindfulness that can permeate other aspects of life. The discipline required in decluttering can also translate into focus and determination in achieving broader life goals. So through the journey of this book, we won't only be clearing out the space, but filling in those empty spaces with lighter dreams and goals that'll drive you forward.

The social side of decluttering cannot be overlooked. It strengthens **relationships and social connections** through teamwork and cooperation among family members as they tackle the decluttering process together. An inviting atmosphere enhances hospitality and also fosters community engagement through donations, helping to stimulate the local economy.

In professional settings, decluttering is a catalyst for **career development**. The habits formed during home organization can elevate your workplace, leading to enhanced productivity and job satisfaction. Clarity gained from a tidy environment can spark innovation and even inspire entrepreneurial ventures.

Decluttering also encourages **spiritual and emotional growth**. It allows for introspection, helping individuals align their environment with their values while offering a therapeutic outlet for healing from trauma.

Beyond that, it frees up precious time for leisure and exploration, creating opportunities for **travel, hobbies, and connection with nature**. You may not be introverted as you think; you may just be overloaded beyond what you imagine. A well-organized home not only facilitates engagement with personal interests but also nurtures a healthier appreciation for the natural world.

The benefits extend to **family dynamics and children** too, as decluttering promotes communication and shared responsibility, offering valuable lessons about charity and environmental stewardship. Finally, let's not forget our furry friends; a decluttered space creates a healthier environment for pets, reducing risks of hazards while potentially benefiting animal welfare through donations.

I could go on and on; the list is endless. I mean, what better thing could happen in your life right now beyond personal freedom? It's everything you'll ever want!

Tool: The Decluttering Checklist

Now, as earlier instructed, keep a bookmark on this list because you'd most likely refer to it every now and then to see how far you've gone in your journey to freedom. You're about to begin a deeply rewarding process and I don't just want you to declutter but to also feel it in your body, your mind, your finances, and your spirit. As you continue this journey, return to this page often and tick off at least seven of the eleven benefits below. Let it serve as your progress tracker and affirmation board.

1. Emotional & Mental Clarity

☐ *I feel less overwhelmed in my space and more at peace in my mind.*

☐ *I've noticed increased focus, creativity, or improved sleep.*

2. Physical Health & Safety

☐ *My space is physically safer, cleaner, and easier to maintain.*

☐ *Decluttering has made way for movement, exercise, or quiet meditation.*

3. Environmental Sustainability

☐ *I've donated, recycled, or responsibly disposed of items.*

☐ I feel more connected to conscious, ethical living.

4. Financial Gains

☐ I've sold or repurposed items I no longer use.

☐ I've noticed I buy less impulsively or save more money.

5. A Peaceful, Inviting Home

☐ I feel prouder to invite people into my space.

☐ My environment reflects who I am and how I want to live.

6. Self-Discovery & Discipline

☐ Decluttering helped me uncover old passions or discover new ones.

☐ I've become more focused, intentional, and goal-driven.

7. Improved Relationships & Community

☐ I've collaborated with loved ones or donated to causes through decluttering.

☐ My space encourages connection and meaningful hospitality.

8. Career & Productivity Boost

☐ My workspace is clearer, and I've become more productive at work.

☐ I've felt more inspired or creative in my career or personal projects.

9. Spiritual & Emotional Healing

☐ Clearing physical clutter has helped me process or release emotional weight.

☐ I feel more aligned with my core values and at peace with my past.

10. More Time & Joyful Living

☐ I have more time and energy for hobbies, travel, or nature.

☐ I feel lighter, freer, and more curious about life again.

11. Family, Children & Pets

☐ Decluttering has improved family teamwork or taught valuable life lessons.

☐ My space is safer and more nurturing for pets and children.

Reflection & Action Step

Now ask yourself:

- Which 2-3 of these benefits have I already begun to notice?
- Which ones do I most desire and how might I prioritize space-making to invite them in?
- Who could I involve in this journey with me?

Keep coming back to this checklist as this is your quiet proof that the exercises are working.

Conclusion

Now that you're all good on the notion of decluttering and making space, alongside the many benefits it brings to you, let's begin the decluttering process, one segment at a time.

Chapter Five
The Hands-On Reset; A Practical Guide to Physical Decluttering

I've always had this thing about me where I got tired of my environment too easily. At first, I thought I was the only one, but there were others who shared the same feeling. It's our one big superpower; we just love new environment. Alright, let's rewind a little – it is no way a superpower. As a matter of fact, it's a terrible headache that follows you all your life. What accompanies you every time is frequent relocation, constant organization and reorganization, stress and longing for outings and tourism.

It was just a matter of time before I got to understand that the physical space dictates a large portion of our existence. I got to figure out that one of the reasons why I got bored or tired of the current space around me was the fact that with time, it all got jumbled up with mess that I would rather escape from than confront. Unfortunately, we don't get to change houses like clothes, and if you're not some stinking rich business mogul, you'll have to start fighting that demon of physical clutter much earlier.

So, nope...you don't need a new house. You need a new relationship with your space.

From the moment you wake up to the moment you shut down your day, the environments around you either support or sabotage your peace. Clutter creates noise, delay, decision fatigue, and emotional drain. But here's the good news: clutter is also one of the few life problems you can literally pick up and throw away.

This chapter gives you real systems; no fluff, no preaching. You'll find strategies, methods, and momentum here. Let's begin right where you are.

Start Where You Stand: Build Momentum in Micro-Wins

You don't need a weekend. You don't need motivation. You don't even need a plan. All you need is to choose one visible surface, and begin.

This is where momentum is born: not in planning, not in perfectionism, but in action. Psychologists call it the *"foot-in-the-door phenomenon"* - when a person agrees to a small request, they're more likely to follow through with a larger one later. The same applies to space. The moment you clear a single corner, your brain registers success and asks for more.

The Power of One Clear Spot

Pick a single small area - a kitchen counter, a coffee table, your bedside stand, your desk. Don't organize or arrange. Simply remove everything and ask:

- What do I actually use every day?
- What belongs here by function?
- What feels like noise or guilt?
- What hasn't moved or served me in months?

Clean the surface. Then return only what is *beautiful, functional, or intentional*. Read those three keywords again.

Soothing Note: *Even a clear bathroom sink can alter how you show up in the morning. A decluttered entry table reduces the chaotic start to your day. A single shelf cleared of junk mail can eliminate stress more than a hundred inbox hacks.*

Why Small Wins Matter

Starting big often leads to decision fatigue, paralysis, or half-finished projects. But a small clear space? That's achievable and visible. And it changes your behavior immediately:

- You feel more in control.
- You clean more easily.
- You stop dumping new things in that area.

• You begin to want this clarity everywhere.

Try This Today:

Choose one of the following and take 20 minutes to clear it completely:

- Your desk surface
- Bathroom counter
- Kitchen island
- Bedside table
- One shelf in your wardrobe
- The top of your refrigerator

Set a timer. Do nothing else. Feel the shift.

Decluttering Methods That Work: Choosing Your Strategy

Decluttering doesn't have to be done randomly. There are actual methods - tested by real people in real spaces - that help you know where to begin, how to make decisions, and how to keep going without giving up halfway. I've tried all these methods and found them very effective.

Think of these strategies like tools in a toolbox. You don't need to use all of them. You can try one and stick with it or combine two that make sense for your lifestyle. The point is to find a method that works with your energy, your goals, and the kind of space you're trying to clean up.

These are the conventional established methods you may find around or hear from friends and my interpretations of these methods to create a clearer understanding for you.

The KonMari Method: Tidy by Category, Not by Room

The KonMari Method was developed by Marie Kondo, a Japanese organizing expert and author of *The Life-Changing Magic of Tidying Up*. Her approach became a global sensation because it encouraged people to only keep things that "spark joy."

But what does that mean, practically?

Here's how the KonMari Method works:

a. You tidy by category, not by location

Most people clean room by room. KonMari suggests cleaning by **category** instead - so instead of "clean the bedroom," you'd start with "clothes" and gather every piece of clothing from the house into one spot. This helps you see the full volume of what you own. The five main categories are:

1. Clothes
2. Books
3. Papers
4. Komono (miscellaneous items like kitchen stuff, tools, make-up, electronics)
5. Sentimental items (photos, letters, gifts)

You tackle each category in that order. The logic is simple: it's easier to make decisions about clothes than it is about love letters or baby pictures. Starting with the easier items builds your decision-making confidence.

b. You hold each item and ask, "Does this spark joy?"

Yes, it might sound odd at first. But the question is really about how your body reacts to something. Do you feel good using or wearing this? Do you feel neutral or even weighed down by it?

If the answer isn't a clear yes, you let it go. Not with guilt, but with gratitude. A quick thank you and then it goes into the discard pile.

This method ensures you are surrounded only by things that actually serve you or make you feel good.

c. Everything has its place

Once you've decluttered by category, KonMari encourages you to store each item where it "lives." Clothes get folded in drawers vertically so you can see each piece. Books go on shelves in a way that allows them to breathe. Containers are reused and nothing is shoved under the bed unless it truly belongs there.

Why it works:

- It forces you to face how much you own.
- It gives you a clear order to follow, which removes guesswork.
- It strengthens your ability to make decisions quickly and honestly.
- It puts emotion into the process in a healthy way.

What to watch out for:

- It can feel overwhelming at the beginning, especially if you own a lot.
- The emotional connection to items can slow you down.
- It requires commitment - you need a few uninterrupted hours or a weekend to go deep.

But for many people, KonMari has been the breakthrough method that helped them finally let go of what no longer serves them and create a space that feels lighter, clearer, and more personal.

The Four-Box Technique: Simple Sorting for Every Room

The Four-Box Technique is exactly what it sounds like: a practical way to declutter using just four boxes (or bins, baskets, bags, anything you have on hand so don't be too quick to rule it out because of the absence of boxes). It's not fancy, and that's the beauty of it. You can use it in any room, at any time, with whatever time or energy you have.

This method is especially helpful if you don't want to overthink things or get stuck wondering what to do with each item. The boxes guide your decisions.

Here's how it works:

You label four boxes (or piles) as follows:

1. **Keep**

2. **Donate**

3. **Throw Away**

4. **Relocate (although some add "sell" to the boxes but I prefer this)**

Let's break each one down.

a. Keep – Things that you genuinely use or love

If you pick something up and it's something you still use, need, or truly enjoy having around, it goes in the Keep box. But here's the catch: don't keep something just because you might need it someday. Be honest with yourself. If it's useful, beautiful, or meaningful, and you actually engage with it, then it deserves to stay.

b. Donate – Still good, just not for you anymore

These are the items in good condition that you simply don't need. Maybe it's a sweater you haven't worn in two years or an extra blender you didn't even realize you had. Somebody else could get real use from it. This box gives you a chance to release clutter with purpose, knowing someone else might benefit from what no longer fits your life.

c. Throw Away – Broken, expired, worn out

Some things are just... done. Worn-out shoes, expired skincare, broken gadgets you swore you'd fix but haven't touched in three years. If it's not worth fixing, giving, or keeping, then it's time to let it go. Don't guilt yourself over it. Just be real. If it's not functional, it goes.

d. Relocate – It belongs somewhere else in your home

You'll always find things that are in the wrong spot: kitchen scissors in your bathroom drawer, books scattered in the pantry, chargers in a sock basket. These aren't exactly clutter, more like misplaced stuff. Instead of running back and forth each time, toss them into the Relocate box and return them to their proper places when you're done.

Why it works:

- It's straightforward. No emotional deep-dives needed.

- It gives you clear action steps for every item.

- It's flexible (you can literally do it in a drawer or an entire house).

- It builds momentum fast. You'll start seeing results within minutes.

What to watch out for:

- Don't skip boxes. It's tempting to create a fifth pile: "I don't know." Resist that. Force yourself to choose.

- The "Keep" box can grow quickly if you're not careful. Be mindful. Just because something is familiar doesn't mean it deserves space.

The Four-Box Technique is excellent for people who get overwhelmed by too many rules. If you want to keep things simple and get things done without over-complicating it, this method is a solid place to begin.

The 12-12-12 Challenge: A Quick Reset When You're Short on Time

The 12-12-12 Challenge is one of the most approachable and fast-paced decluttering methods out there. It was popularized by Joshua Becker of *Becoming Minimalist,* and it's perfect for people who feel stuck or overwhelmed and just need to get going. There's no fuss, no paralysis.

This method is exactly what the name implies: a small, focused challenge where you find...

- 12 items to throw away,

- 12 items to donate, and

- 12 items to return to their proper place.

That's it. 36 items, sorted in one short burst.

How to do it:

1.   Pick a room or space: your bedroom, your kitchen, your home office.

2.   Start moving through it and pull out 12 items in each of the three categories.

3.   Work fast. Don't overthink. Trust your first instinct.

Here are some notes on the selecting of your items:

a. Throw Away – Outdated, broken, useless

Find 12 things that have no place in your life anymore. This could be expired food in the pantry, old receipts, broken chargers, empty lotion bottles, stretched-out socks - whatever's past its prime.

b. Donate – Good stuff you just don't use

Next, look for 12 items that are still in decent condition but aren't serving you anymore. Old bags, unused mugs, clothes that don't fit or match your style, unopened gifts, duplicate tools. These are the things that someone else might appreciate more than you do.

c. Return to Place – Items that are just out of order

Last, find 12 items that belong somewhere else. This is your reset group: shoes in the living room that belong in the closet, chargers left on the floor, notebooks stacked in the kitchen. It's surprising how much order comes back into a space just by returning a few things where they belong.

Why it works:

• It's fast. You can finish a round in 10–20 minutes.

• It's energizing. You feel immediate relief after doing it.

• It removes decision fatigue. You have a number to hit - nothing more.

• It builds rhythm. You can repeat it daily or weekly.

What to watch out for:

- It's not a deep-clean. This method is more about momentum than perfection.

- If you try it and can't find 12 of each item, don't force it. Go with what you can and try again later.

- It can become a fun game, but don't lose sight of the goal: clearing what no longer serves you.

The 12-12-12 Challenge is perfect for weekends, evenings, or any time you feel the itch to declutter but don't want to commit to a massive overhaul. Think of it as a reset button for your space. Do it regularly, and over time, you'll see big results from small, consistent actions.

The Minimalism Game: A Bold, Day-by-Day Countdown

If you like a bit of structure mixed with challenge, *The Minimalism Game* might be the one that sticks. Created by Joshua Fields Millburn and Ryan Nicodemus (a.k.a. The Minimalists), this method turns decluttering into a 30-day competition against yourself or others.

Dang!

It's simple:

On Day 1, get rid of 1 item.

On Day 2, get rid of 2 items.

Day 3? 3 items.

All the way to Day 30, where you'll let go of 30 items. Or 31 items for 31 days.

That's 465 items gone in one month. Yep - 465.

How it works:

- Start on the first of any month (or just any Monday if you prefer).

- Each day, declutter the number of items that corresponds to that day.

- These items can be *donated, trashed, sold, or given away* - as long as they leave your space.

- You can do this alone, or challenge a friend or partner to keep pace.

Tips for success:

- **Create a staging area.** Have a box or corner where you place all decluttered items before donating or disposing of them.

- **Use your phone.** Snap a daily photo of the items to keep track. It's satisfying to look back at the progress.

- **Start easy.** Begin with the junk drawer or that overflowing kitchen cabinet. Leave the sentimental stuff for later in the month when your decluttering muscles are stronger.

- **Stay flexible.** If you miss a day, don't quit - just catch up the next day or spread those items across the week.

Why it works:

I love this system because you'll build momentum. You ease in with small numbers, and by the time the challenge gets tough, you're in the groove. It's also measurable it gives you have a daily goal. That structure helps fight decision fatigue.

By the end of the month, you'll have trained yourself to look at your belongings more critically. It can be fun, especially if done with someone else - it adds accountability and turns decluttering into a game.

What to watch out for:

- The end of the month can feel intense. Day 27? That's 27 things in one day. But that's where the transformation happens. It pushes you to go beyond surface-level clutter.

• Don't cheat yourself. Throwing out 27 receipts doesn't count. The idea is to let go of meaningful, space-consuming items.

The Minimalism Game is perfect for people who love countdowns, streaks, and challenges. If you're someone who thrives with a goal and enjoys proving something to yourself, this method can make decluttering feel less like a chore and more like a personal victory.

The Ski-Slope Method: Declutter from the Top Down

If you're the type that thrives on flow and visual progress, the Ski-Slope Method might be your perfect match. Like some of the methods I've discussed earlier, it's not much about numbers but more about momentum. Think of it as carving your way down a mountain so you go smooth, strategic, and gravity-assisted. You start high, and you glide lower with purpose.

Yep, you're skiing through your clutter.

Here's the gist:

You begin decluttering at the highest points of your space like top shelves, high cupboards, anything above eye level. Then, like a skier descending a slope, you move to mid-level surfaces (desks, countertops, drawers), and finally end at the base like the floors, under furniture, and ground-level storage.

How it works:

• Pick your "slope" which could be a single room, a closet, or an entire home.

• Start at the top: Remove items from high-up areas that often get ignored or just accumulate dust.

• Work your way down: Tackle mid-levels next, then finish with what's at your feet (literally).

• No backtracking: Resist the urge to jump around. Stay on the slope.

Tips for success:

• Use gravity to your advantage. As you pull things down from higher areas, you'll naturally create space to sort below.

• Bring a step stool or ladder. It helps you fully access the top zones and gives you a reason not to avoid them.

• Keep a donation box close. That way, you don't have to keep going up and down the slope to drop stuff off.

• Clear as you go. Wipe down those newly exposed surfaces to really feel the refresh.

Why it works:

I like this method because it mimics how our eyes (and brains) scan a space. High-up clutter gets ignored until it doesn't. By starting there, you shift the energy of a room early. And as you move lower, things literally lighten up. Each level feels like a checkpoint, giving you mini-wins without needing to overthink categories or item counts.

Plus, there's something calming about working with gravity. It feels like the room is naturally settling into place.

What to watch out for:

• The temptation to stash. As you bring things down, don't just relocate them to another shelf or pile. You should make real decisions.

• Overwhelm on big slopes. If you're working in a large area, divide it into smaller sections (like "ski runs") so you don't burn out halfway.

• Skipping the floor. It's easy to stop once eye-level looks good. But the magic really happens when you clear the base.

The Ski-Slope Method is ideal if you crave calm over chaos, and love seeing a room transform in layers. It's great for visual learners, big-picture thinkers, or anyone who wants to reset their space with a sense of flow and not just the use of force.

The Packing Party: Unpack Only What You Truly Need

If you've ever wondered what life would feel like with just the essentials, the Packing Party might be your wake-up call. I tried this once, although it worked best when we had an actual party; that is, when I was in the midst of friends in our early youthful days and as the session for resumption drew by, we just saw the need to clear out our mess. This bold decluttering method flips the script: instead of deciding what to get rid of, you pretend you're moving and then only "unpack" what you use. Sounds extreme? It kind of is. But that's what makes it work.

Now, imagine you're moving out today. You grab some boxes and pack up everything in your home... yes, everything. Every book, every spoon, every throw pillow. Now your home looks like you just moved in... but you're not going anywhere.

Over the next few weeks, you only unpack the things you actually use. Everything else just sits in the box. In no time, the clutter will be left in the box.

How it works:

• Get your supplies: Boxes, tape, labels like a real move.

• Box it all up: Pack every single item in your space. Clothes, décor, dishes, the works.

• Live your life: When you need something, take it out and put it back in its proper place after use.

• Set a time limit: After 21 or 30 days (or whatever you choose), whatever's still in boxes... probably doesn't belong in your life. Trash it!

To make the best of this process, label the boxes: not with the contents, but with the room or category (e.g. "Bedroom – Misc"). Be as honest as you can be. Don't unpack just because you might need something someday. Only grab what you genuinely use. Also, start small if needed: try this method on a single closet, room, or drawer before committing to your whole house. And of all, don't do this alone. It's more fun if you live with others so you can make it a group challenge. Each person gets their own boxes and rules.

Why it works:

The experience I had with the Packing Party was a lovely one because it removed decision fatigue. You're not standing there holding an old sweater asking, "Should I keep this?" You just... don't unpack it unless it proves its worth in your actual, daily life.

It's also incredibly revealing. You realise how little you really need and how much you're holding onto out of habit, guilt, or inertia. Plus, it turns your home into a fresh, open space. A bit like moving into a new apartment, minus the van rental. So you feel like you've moved to a new home subconsciously.

What to watch out for:

It's not subtle. Your home will look like a warehouse at first. Be prepared for that visual shift and bear in mind that it's temporary. Also, you need time and energy to pack up properly. This is a front-loaded method, but the payoff is big.

Sentimental items need care. Maybe have a separate "memory box" so you're not unpacking your kid's first drawing just to find a can opener. The Packing Party is for people who want to hit reset. It's ideal if you've tried decluttering bit by bit with little success, and you're ready for a radical, all-in approach. It's less about what you're willing to let go of and more about discovering what truly deserves to stay.

Room by Room Deep Dive

Let's comb through thoroughly like we've never done before:

Living Room: Tech/Media Purge & Décor Rethink

Start by auditing electronic clutter: discard obsolete chargers, controllers, and gadgets that haven't been used in six months (a "tech graveyard" audit).

Keep only necessary devices and neatly corral cords (use cable clips or a cord box) so they don't dominate the space. Rethink décor with an eye for simplicity: aim to let shelves and surfaces "breathe." Avoid overfilling them; leaving even 25% of a shelf empty creates an airy, curated look and prevents visual overload.

Opt for a few meaningful decor pieces instead of many knick-knacks. Store or donate excess magazines and books, keeping only favourites (digital subscriptions can replace stacks of magazines).

Use closed storage (like baskets or cabinets) to hide everyday items when not in use, maintaining a calm vibe. In short, purge tech clutter and curate decor so the living room feels open and inviting, not a tangle of wires or a jumble of objects.

Kitchen & Pantry: "Breathable" Kitchenware & Food Declutter

In the kitchen, focus on freeing space and ensuring everything stored is truly needed. Purge duplicates and rarely-used gadgets: you likely don't need four spatulas or that bread maker collecting dust. Keep versatile tools and donate the rest.

Streamline dishware to a sensible set for your household (plus a few extras for guests). Next, tackle the pantry: clear it out completely and toss expired or stale foods – these waste space and add "friction" when trying to cook.

Donate unopened non-perishables you won't use (check expiry dates first). Group what remains into logical categories (grains, snacks, baking, etc.) for easy access.

Aim to store foods in breathable or transparent containers: for example, use baskets or ventilated bins for produce like potatoes and onions, and clear canisters for dry goods. This not only preserves freshness but also lets you see inventory at a glance (preventing over-buying).

Finally, reclaim counter space – stow away infrequently used appliances to give your kitchen "breathing room." A decluttered, open countertop makes daily cooking and cleaning much easier. By paring down cookware and keeping only regularly used, multi-functional items, your kitchen will feel more spacious and efficient.

Bathroom: Meds, Beauty Products & Linens

Bathrooms accumulate expired and excess items, so do a critical sweep. Discard expired medications, sunscreens, and makeup – using them can be ineffective or even unsafe. (Follow local guidelines for safe medication disposal, like dropping off at a pharmacy, rather than tossing in the trash.)

Pare down grooming products: if you have half-used bottles, you don't actually like, let them go. Similarly, toss old or spoiled cosmetics and skincare to reduce clutter and protect your skin. Streamline to the daily basics plus a few favourites.

Next, tackle linens: pull out any towels that are frayed, musty, or stained – these are less absorbent and hygienic anyway. Keep a reasonable number of good towels (two per person, perhaps) and donate or repurpose the rest (animal shelters often welcome old towels).

Store backup toiletries and cleaning supplies in clear bins so you can see what you have (avoiding inadvertently buying duplicates).

Finally, remove excess packaging – items like soap, cotton swabs, or dental floss can be decanted into labelled containers or drawers to cut visual clutter. You'll find your morning and bedtime routines calmer in a space with tidy drawers, a curated skincare shelf, and only fresh, fluffy towels at hand.

Bedroom & Wardrobe: Customize the KonMari Method + The "Four-Corner" Rule

Bring order to your bedroom by decluttering with strategies that blend Marie Kondo's joy-centric approach with practical customization. Empty out your wardrobe or closet onto the bed and pick up each clothing item, deciding whether to keep, donate, or toss. Keep only what you truly need or deeply love wearing. This echoes the KonMari "spark joy" criterion, but also consider fit and lifestyle. For example, an expensive dress that doesn't fit or suit you can go, even if it once sparked joy. As you edit, be mindful of emotional attachments; try to focus less on the guilt of letting things go, and more on the benefits (more space, a wardrobe that "serves" you daily).

To avoid overwhelm, apply the "four-corner rule" when tidying the room itself: divide the bedroom into four zones (for instance, each corner or section of the room) and tackle one area at a time, fully completing it before moving on. This method keeps you focused and prevents half-finished piles everywhere.

In the closet, group remaining clothes by category (and even by colour) when you put them back e.g. hang dresses together, shirts together, etc., for visibility. Use smart storage like drawer dividers and under-bed bins for off-season clothing or extra bedding. You can also rotate seasonal clothes: pack winter coats away during summer and vice versa, so your closet only contains current-season garments (making it easier to see and use everything).

One more tip to customize KonMari: if the strict "joy" test feels too extreme, impose a practical rule. For example, the 1-year rule (if you haven't worn it in a year, strongly consider letting it go) or the Rule of 4 (each kept item should be versatile enough to wear in at least 4 different outfits). By blending sentimental consideration with functionality, you'll end up with a bedroom that is cozy and personalized, but also free of excess.

Workspace/Home Office: The Zen Strategy – Gather, Sort, Purge, Organize

Treat your workspace declutter like a mini-project. First, gather every item from your desk, drawers, and office shelves into one area. Having it all in sight forces a reckoning with how much stuff has accumulated.

Next, sort items into categories (e.g. papers, office supplies, tech devices, etc.) and immediately set aside obvious trash or duplicates. Then purge ruthlessly: throw out junk mail, outdated documents (shred if sensitive), dried-up pens, and donate electronics or books you no longer need. Only keep what is either essential for work or truly inspiring to you.

Finally, organize what's left into a logical system. Give everything a designated "home" in your office: use file folders for important papers, drawer organizers for supplies, and shelves or bins for books and equipment. Aim for a clean desktop with only daily-use tools on it. This four-step approach (gather, sort, purge, organize) is a systematic way to tackle any area as it ensures you don't skip the critical editing (purge) phase before trying to rearrange things.

As you reorganize, also label files or storage containers for easy retrieval (e.g. label cords or chargers in a tech basket). By using this Zen Strategy, you'll create a workspace where your mind can focus, with only the tools you need at your fingertips and nothing unnecessary to distract you.

Entryway, Garage & Storage Areas: Functional Entryway & Seasonal Reset

These transitional and storage spaces need decluttering love too. For the entryway, adopt a "less is more" mindset because this area is your home's first impression and a functional drop-zone.

Assign a clear purpose: an entryway is for coming-and-going essentials – keys, shoes, coats, maybe mail – and nothing beyond that. Remove any items that don't serve that daily transition. (As professional organizers say, the entry isn't a storage room, it's a "transition zone".)

Set up hooks or a coat rack for jackets, a bowl or rack for keys and sunglasses, and perhaps a small bench or shelf for shoes and bags. Keep only current season items here: for example, don't clog the hallway with every coat you own. Store out-of-season outerwear elsewhere because leaving your heavy parka hanging by the door all summer just wastes valuable space. One idea is to have a basket or bin in the entry closet dedicated to off-season gear, rotated as the weather changes.

Also implement a simple routine: each evening or once a week, reset the entry. Put stray shoes back in closets, recycle junk mail, etc. In the garage and storage areas, plan a seasonal declutter sweep at least a couple of times a year. Garages often become dumping grounds for things we "might need someday." Instead, treat your garage like an extension of your home: group sports equipment in one zone, tools in another, decorations in another. As you declutter, donate or toss things you didn't use in the last year (that old camping gear or busted lawn chair).

A seasonal reset means at the end of each season, you reevaluate and store things accordingly: for example, as winter ends, store holiday decor and snow shovels toward the back, and bring spring/summer items (gardening tools, bicycles) to the forefront. Likewise, when fall arrives, rotate again. This ensures you're not perpetually working around items that aren't even in season.

For long-term storage, use clear bins and label them ("Winter Clothes," "Halloween Decor") so you can find things when needed.

Lastly, remember garages can accumulate hazardous materials (old paint, antifreeze, etc.). Identify those during your declutter and dispose of them properly (most cities have hazardous waste drop-off events; never put them in regular trash). An orderly entryway saves you from morning stress (no frantic searches for keys!), and a decluttered garage means you can actually park the car or find the toolbox without tripping over clutter.

Taming Paper & Digital Overflow

If you're the type that deals with hardcopy writing most times, much like I am, you're prone to a paper disaster. Let's get that aspect sorted out:

Sort Paper into Keep / Shred / Digitize

Paper clutter can overwhelm if not triaged. Begin by gathering all loose papers (from countertops, drawers, bags) into one stack and then classify each item into one of three categories:

1) **Keep (important originals)** – like birth certificates, passports, property deeds, or certain legal documents that you must retain in physical form;

2) **Shred/Toss** – junk mail, old bills or statements you don't need, expired coupons, etc., especially anything with personal info should go through the shredder;

3) **Digitize (then discard)** – documents you don't need physically but want to save information from (for example, tax returns from a few years ago, medical records, or sentimental papers like kids' artwork). For this third pile, scan them with a scanner or a scanner app on your phone, back up the files, and then recycle or shred the paper copy. Adopting this "scan and toss" habit can drastically reduce paper volume. In fact, experts note that the vast majority of old paperwork can be thrown out once digitized. Only a small handful of papers with original signatures or seals truly need to be kept in file.

Set up a simple filing system for the papers you do keep. For instance, use a small file box or cabinet with labelled folders for key categories: e.g. Insurance, Taxes, House, Medical, etc. Aim for a system that is logically organized, easy to access, and has a bit of room to grow. Don't overcomplicate it; the simpler and more intuitive, the more likely you'll maintain it.

Finally, handle incoming papers immediately when possible: sort mail as soon as it comes (recycle junk mail, file what's important, and set aside any "action items" like bills to pay in a designated spot). By continuously funnelling papers into these categories (keep, shred, or scan), you prevent piles from building up. Over time, strive to go increasingly paperless – opt for e-statements, digital note-taking, etc., to keep new paper to a minimum.

Set Up Simple Folder Systems (Physical)

Good organization systems are the backbone of staying clutter-free. Design systems that are simple, logical, and consistent. For physical papers as mentioned, a small filing cabinet with clearly labelled folders is essential.

A well-designed folder system (whether manila folders or digital directories which we'll be discussing in later chapters) saves you time and frustration. It also ensures that when new papers or files come in, you know exactly where to put them, meaning clutter is far less likely to accumulate in the first place. Ultimately, a simple system you actually use is better than a "perfect" complex system that you abandon. Set up something that makes sense to you, and then maintain it with small, regular habits (like filing documents immediately, or doing a quick digital file clean-up monthly).

Sentimental Items Strategy

Sentimental clutter is the toughest to tackle because of the emotions attached. The goal here is to honor important memories without keeping every object associated with them.

Manage Keepsakes Mindfully (Memory Boxes & Photos)

Start by designating one or a few "memory boxes." These are containers (like a nice bin or chest) where you store your most treasured keepsakes – letters, heirlooms, childhood souvenirs, etc. Limiting yourself to the space of the box forces selectivity: when the box is full, you must remove something if you want to add a new item. As you sort through sentimental things, it may help to tell the story of the item; reminisce about why it's meaningful.

Often, you'll find that the story or memory is what you truly value, not the physical item itself. In such cases, you can take a photograph of the item (or scan letters and kids' artwork) and then let the item go, knowing you've preserved the memory digitally. Writing a short note about the item's significance and storing that with the photo can also capture the sentiment (for example, "This was Grandma's vase that she used every New Year's. It reminds me of her smile"). As decluttering expert Courtney Carver notes, *"Your heart doesn't want to hold on to stuff, it just wants the love and story behind it."* This realization can make it easier to release objects that are just gathering dust.

Another tip: display a few cherished items instead of squirreling everything away. Curate a small "memory shelf" or section of a bookcase where you showcase, say, 5–10 sentimental items that make you happy. By spotlighting a limited number, you give those items respect and attention, rather than diluting the sentiment in a cluttered pile of dozens of trinkets. You can frame a couple of your favourite family photos (rather than keeping hundreds of prints in a box), or keep one baby outfit that meant the most and donate the rest. It's also helpful to differentiate true treasures from guilt keepsakes. You might be holding onto your late aunt's entire tea set out of guilt, even though you never use it. Maybe keep one teacup that reminds you of her and donate the rest to someone who will use it. Memory preservation alternatives like creating a digital photo-book of a collection, or making a quilt from old t-shirts, can transform clutter into accessible memories.

Finally, give yourself permission to let go in stages. You don't have to purge all sentimental items in one go. You can declutter in rounds, each time parting with a few things as you feel ready.

Try the "10-Item Memory Shelf" to Spotlight What Matters

This is a practical exercise for limiting sentimental items is to create a 10-Item Memory Shelf. Select a shelf or small display area in your home and choose up to ten cherished items to live there. These could be a mix of framed photos, mementos, awards, travel souvenirs, whatever items instantly spark joy and represent your most valued memories or accomplishments. This doesn't mean you only own ten sentimental things total, but it does mean only ten are out on display at once. Here, I usually include a rotational system, where if you want to introduce a new item to the shelf, you remove something else to storage (or decide it's time to let it go entirely).

The "10-item" number is arbitrary, of course. You can choose a number that fits your space (for some it might be five, for others maybe one per family member). I began with ten though.

The key factor applied here is the principle of deliberate limitation. It forces you to discern which pieces mean the most. For example, instead of cluttering your living room with dozens of family knick-knacks, you might display a top ten: perhaps your grandfather's pocket watch, your wedding photo, a shell from that special beach trip, etc. This also makes it easier to maintain as dusting 10 items on a shelf is far easier than managing 50 scattered around the house.

Additionally, involve the family in this if you live with others: maybe each person gets to pick a couple of items for the memory shelf, which is a lovely way to share stories with each other. When you notice an item on the shelf no longer tugs your heartstrings as it used to, that could be a signal that you're ready to let it move on (freeing a slot for something else meaningful).

The memory shelf concept aligns with the idea that "less is more" when it comes to sentimental displays. A few truly special items have a greater emotional impact than a clutter of many. By spotlighting a limited selection, you consciously celebrate those memories. Over time, you might find that you don't miss the items that never make it out of storage, which can give you confidence to declutter them permanently.

Collaborative Decluttering

Decluttering is much easier (and even fun) when everyone in the household gets involved. If you live with family or roommates, try these collaborative approaches:

Schedule Shared Declutter Sessions

Set aside a time (say, a Saturday morning each month or a "clean-up day") when everyone works on decluttering together. This creates a team atmosphere and a bit of accountability. You can focus on common areas or each tackle personal spaces simultaneously. Play upbeat music and perhaps order a pizza after as a reward. Seeing each other declutter can be motivating (and no one feels singled out).

Turn Decluttering into a Game

For kids especially, gamify the process. One idea is the "15-minute declutter challenge" – set a timer and see who can find 10 items to put in the donate box the fastest. Or a scavenger hunt: "find five things in your room you haven't used in months." One mom shared that she dumped all her kids' toys on the floor and gave each child a box, telling them they could keep only what fit in their box – the kids actually thought it was fun, like a puzzle, and the whole toy purge was done in under 2 hours.

You can also use decision games like "Would You Rather?" Hold up an item and ask the child (or roommate), "Would you rather keep this, or have the space it frees up (or the money it could sell for)?" Sometimes phrasing it that way sparks a rethink. Or try the classic coin flip for items everyone's indecisive about; heads you keep for now, tails it goes; it adds a light-hearted luck element.

Establish Donation Rituals

Making donation a positive, even celebrated act can help those reluctant to let go. Perhaps start a tradition that each season, the family fills one box of items to donate to charity together, then you all go to the donation center and maybe get ice cream after. I know of a family that does a monthly "give-away day" where each person chooses one of their possessions to donate to someone less fortunate. It becomes a lesson in generosity as well as decluttering. You could also involve kids by letting them choose where to donate (e.g. books to the library, toys to a children's hospital, clothes to a shelter) so they feel the impact of giving.

Another idea is the "one-in-one-out game" played collectively: if a new toy or gadget comes into the home, the family as a whole finds one old item to leave. It encourages everyone to think about balance, not just accumulation.

Shared Rules & Zones

Agree on some household rules, like "No clutter on the dining table; it's an eating space, not storage," or create a family drop zone by the entry where everyone's backpack, purse, etc. goes instead of all over the house. Post a friendly reminder chart if needed (especially with kids; stickers for putting away their things each day, etc.)

What Goes Where? Disposal Strategies

Now, as much as you badly want to get all those mess out of your house, you have to do so responsibly. Here's how to handle different categories:

1. Donate usable items to local charities or community groups.

Clothes in good condition can go to organizations like Goodwill, Salvation Army, or local shelters. Many communities have specific drives e.g. a women's shelter for professional clothing, or a children's hospital thrift store for toys. Books can often be donated to libraries or little free libraries, and kitchenware to refugee resettlement organizations or community centers. When donating, be considerate: donate items that are clean and functional. If something is truly junk or broken, don't offload it on charities (they then have to pay to dispose of it).

2. Upcycle or repurpose creatively for items that aren't easily donated.

Old towels and blankets, for instance, can become pet bedding (animal shelters will gladly take them) or cleaning rags. A dresser with a broken drawer might be upcycled into a TV stand or taken by a DIY enthusiast. You can list it for free online for someone who likes to refurbish furniture. Upcycling can also mean breaking items down: maybe reuse the fabric from sentimental t-shirts to make a quilt, or convert glass jars into storage containers rather than tossing them.

3.   Recycle everything you can.

This goes beyond just paper and cans. Check your city's recycling programs. Many places accept e-waste (old electronics, cables) on certain days, and big retailers often have bins for recycling batteries, plastic bags, or ink cartridges. When decluttering paperwork, recycle the paper after shredding the sensitive stuff. Old appliances or metal items can often be picked up by scrap metal recyclers.

4.   Hazardous materials need special care

Things like paints, chemicals, automotive fluids, pesticides, certain cleaners, old medications, and electronics contain components that should never go in regular trash. Look up your local municipality's guidelines. Most have Household Hazardous Waste (HHW) drop-off events or centers. For example, used motor oil can often go to an auto shop or designated site, old paint can sometimes be taken to a recycling center or a community paint swap, and expired medications can be turned in at pharmacies or police stations on drug take-back days. Likewise, old electronics (TVs, computers, phones) often have e-cycling programs. Sometimes the store you bought it from will take it back, or the city has an e-waste drop-off. It's worth the extra effort: hazardous waste in landfills can leak toxins into soil and water, and electronics contain valuable materials that can be reclaimed. Many communities now also recycle textiles (for cloth too worn to donate, there are "textile recycling" bins or pickup services. They repurpose fibres into insulation, rags, etc.).

5.   Sell Online: Second-Hand Tips, Pricing, Shipping

Some items you've decluttered might fetch some cash in the second-hand market, which is a nice bonus and encourages reuse. Whether you use Facebook Marketplace, eBay, Poshmark, or Craigslist, simply choose what works best for you, present your items well, write a good description, price it right and be smart with your shipping and pickup.

If you have many low-value items (like lots of kids' clothes or books), consider bundling them as a lot ("whole box of toddler clothes, $20"). It's faster than individual sales. Always be clear about condition; if something is for parts or has a defect, say so up front. For fragile items, pack carefully and maybe require the buyer to pay for insurance if shipping.

Lastly, manage expectations. You likely won't get back what you originally paid (except maybe for rare collectibles), but the goal is to get a fair value while finding your item a new home.

Maintenance for Systems that Stick

Congratulations – you've decluttered and reorganized! Now, the real key is maintaining this new order. Clutter has a way of slowly sneaking back if we don't have routines in place. One of the best habits you can adopt is a weekly 15-Minute Reset.

The Weekly "15 Minute Reset"

The idea is simple: once a week, set a timer for 15 minutes (or 10, or 20 – whatever fits your home size and schedule) and do a quick walk-through of the main living areas to put things back in their designated places. Since everything in your home now has a place (thanks to your decluttering and organizing work), this reset is relatively easy and even meditative. For example, every Sunday evening, you might do a tour: pick up any stray items; the book left on the couch, the shoes by the door, the random coffee mug on the desk – and return them "home."

Monthly Room Check-Ins

In addition to the quick weekly resets, plan a slightly more in-depth monthly check-in for each room. This is a mini-review of the space to ensure everything still has a home and to address any clutter "hot spots" that might be developing. For instance, one weekend a month, take 30-60 minutes to focus on one area. Maybe this month you sweep through the bedrooms, next month the kitchen and pantry, the following month the garage, and so on (or you can do a whole-house walkthrough if you prefer).

This is also the time to rotate or update stored items: for example, a monthly closet check might remind you to bring seasonal clothes forward (swap those heavy coats for the lighter jackets in spring). Use these check-ins to do tiny declutters; the kind of things that take 5 minutes but save grief later, like scanning the fridge for expired items at the end of each month, or going through the mail basket and shredding old paperwork.

Apply the One In, One Out Rule to Stay Grounded

We touched on this above, but it's worth emphasizing as a core maintenance principle: for every new item that comes into your home, make it a habit that one item goes out.

This practice keeps your overall volume of possessions in check, preventing the gradual creep of clutter. It can even become a kind of personal challenge or family game. For example, if you get a new pair of shoes, choose an old pair that's worn out or seldom worn and remove it (donate if in decent shape, or trash if not). Got your kids a new toy? Encourage them to donate one they've outgrown. If you upgrade your blender, let the old one go instead of storing a spare. This rule works especially well for things like clothing, toys, tools, kitchen gadgets – categories where accumulation is common.

Remember: Keep an active donation box somewhere accessible (garage, closet) precisely for this purpose. As soon as you identify an outgoing item, toss it in the box; when the box fills, drop it off at your donation center.

If you ever find the house feeling a bit tight again, just remember to check the inflow: stick to the rule, and you'll stay in control.

Lastly, celebrate how far you've come: maintenance is so much easier than the big purge was! A tidy 15 minutes here, a quick one-out when something comes in, and you preserve a home that truly supports your life – functional, flowing, and filled only with what adds value for you and your family.

Chapter Six
The Headspace Detox: Attaining Mental Organization and Clarity

Going into the part of the brain is a whole new thing, so you shouldn't be so surprised when I use the word "detox." Detox and declutter are used interchangeably in most cases, but for me, I find a little-tiny difference between them.

Clutter seems more physical for me; like that mess that we can see unfolding right before us. Toxins happen to be more inward; the harmful substance we cannot see but feel and experience within our bodies. I've used these terms these ways for so long that they both stuck that way, although till today, other writers or platforms may still use them interchangeably. When it comes to the mental health, I see harmful toxins within our brains, and trust me, there is a desperate need to flush these out. Let me give you an instance.

Have you ever had 37 tabs open in your brain at once?

Me too.

It was a Wednesday - the kind of midweek that feels like it's chewing on both ends. I had back-to-back meetings, dinner to think about, and a relentless reel of thoughts running in the background: *Did I reply to that email? What was that thing I needed to do for Mum? Why haven't I started that project?*

At one point, I found myself staring blankly at the kettle, holding my phone in one hand and a fork in the other. I wasn't cooking or texting. I wasn't even doing anything meaningful. I was just... buffering. Like a browser stuck on a spinning wheel of "loading."

Yep, the way you read it now is exactly how mental clutter feels.

Your mental space has become so cluttered, you can't hear yourself think. And you'll miss you. Mental clutter is that sneaky. It builds gradually with things like an unchecked to-do list here, an emotional hangover there, the never-ending input of content, expectations, decisions and then, it overtakes.

In this chapter, we're going to clear the cobwebs. Think of this as a mental spring cleaning where we learn not only how to offload the mess but also how to create a structure that keeps it from building up again. You'll learn practical, science-backed techniques to lighten the load, protect your mind's clarity, and finally reclaim the kind of stillness that fuels direction.

Mental Decluttering Techniques That Actually Work

Unlike the physical clutters, we may not be able to set four boxes before us to declutter the mind. It takes such unique processes as both types of clutter are distinctively different. You can have a clear physical space but still be tormented by mental clutter. Most draining clutter is often invisible: racing thoughts, unspoken worries, endless to-dos, emotional loops we haven't closed.

Mental clutter has real effects. According to psychologists, too many open cognitive loops (those "I'll deal with it later" thoughts) can cause decision fatigue, stress, and even low-grade anxiety. However, you don't have to live in your head like it's a hoarder's flat. There are simple, research-supported techniques that can help you offload, organize, and clear space for clarity and creativity.

The Brain Dump Method

There's something deeply relieving about getting it all out; not pretty, not polished, just out.

Think of a brain dump as a mental exhale. It's a raw, unfiltered release of everything that's swirling around in your mind. It doesn't need to take an order or a form of arrangement. All you need is you, a pen, and a blank page (or a notes app, if that's your thing though I'd prefer paper here).

Cognitive science shows that we have limited mental bandwidth, what's known as **working memory**. When it's full of unsorted thoughts ("I need to call Aunt Janet... I should finally fix the printer... Did I lock the door?"), we get overwhelmed. The brain dump clears those thoughts from your internal RAM and stores them externally - where they can be seen, sorted, and dealt with later; what we call a to-do list.

A 2021 article from Wide Lens Leadership highlights this practice as one of the fastest ways to reduce cognitive clutter and improve decision-making clarity.

How To Do a Brain Dump

1.   Set a Timer: 5 to 10 minutes. That's all it takes.

2.   Choose Your Medium: Journal, notebook, notes app; whatever feels natural.

3.   Write Without Editing: Let your thoughts pour out in a stream-of-consciousness flow. No structure, no categories, no overthinking.

4.   Include Everything: To-dos, random thoughts, feelings, questions, reminders, worries. If it's in your head, it goes on the page.

5.   Stop When the Timer Dings: Don't push it. Let it feel like a release, not another task.

After the Dump

Once you've finished, take a moment to breathe. You don't have to do anything with what you wrote, at least not right away. But if you want to take it a step further, you can glance over it and highlight:
   • Action items (something to schedule or complete)
   • Emotional threads (something to journal or talk through)
   • Rubbish (stuff you can immediately discard)

The 2-Minute Rule for Thoughts

"If it'll take less than two minutes, do it now!"

That's it.

A deceptively simple rule; one that's been echoed in productivity circles, most famously by David Allen in *Getting Things Done*. But beyond task lists, this rule becomes a mental clarity tool when applied to thoughts.

We all have mental clutter that doesn't actually need deep processing; it just needs a moment of action.

Think of it this way:

- "I need to confirm that appointment." → Text them.
- "I should refill my water bottle." → Stand up, go.
- "I forgot to send that link." → Open, send, done.

These thoughts hang around because we keep postponing what could be cleared in seconds. And while they seem harmless, over time they add up, crowding your focus, dragging your energy...

Here's how to use the 2-Minute Rule for Mental Clarity:

1.   Notice the quick-thoughts: They tend to show up disguised as "I'll do that later."
2.   Ask: Can I finish this in under two minutes?
3.   If yes, act immediately. If not, park it somewhere you trust like a list, a planner, your task app.

Why it works:

It clears the cache. Like deleting the mental pop-ups before they multiply. Every quick action is a small mental reset. You feel lighter, clearer not because your to-do list vanished, but because your mental drag reduced.

Mind Mapping for Clarity

Sometimes, our minds feel messy because we're trying to think in straight lines when our thoughts were never meant to be linear.

That's where mind mapping comes in.

Unlike lists or bullet points, mind maps reflect how the brain actually works through associations, connections and clusters. At any given moment, we're thinking not in order, but in sparks: one idea leads to another, and another and it goes on. A mind map doesn't try to force order prematurely but instead, it welcomes the mess, then gently gives it structure.

Picture this: you're overwhelmed with everything you need to handle this week. We're talking work, family, health, personal projects. You sit down to make a list, but it's endless and oddly stressful. That's because your list is trying to stack thoughts that were never meant to sit on top of each other. Mind mapping lets you spread them out.

You begin by placing a central word in the middle of a page - something broad like "This Week" or "Mental Load."

From there, you draw branches: maybe one says "Work," another says "Home," and another "Me."

Under "Work" you scribble meetings, deadlines, loose ends. Under "Home," you add errands, family stuff, bills. "Me" holds your quiet dreams: journal, stretch, breathe.

Before long, your mental fog starts to part because mind mapping externalises the chaos. It turns the cloud of your thoughts into something visible and manageable. Researchers in cognitive psychology suggest that visual processing helps with clarity and memory retention because when you see your thoughts laid out spatially, you begin to understand them more deeply.

It's also deeply personal. Your mind map is yours alone. It is imperfect, scribbly and raw. It doesn't have to look pretty. It just has to make sense to you.

And that's the real gift of mind mapping that made me love it dearly: it's self-connection. You're no longer just reacting to the noise in your head but you're gently stepping back, observing, and choosing your direction with intention. Because when your mind can see where it's going, the rest of you tends to follow.

Thought Curation

Not every thought deserves a seat at your table.

One of the most powerful forms of mental clarity doesn't come from doing more, but from deciding less. Let that ring.

What I mean by this is curating your thoughts which is intentionally choosing which ideas are worth keeping, which are noise, and which are just passing through.

We often assume every thought is equal, that if something shows up in our mind, we must entertain it. But imagine if your physical home worked that way. Imagine letting in every visitor, collecting every flyer, keeping every empty box. You'd be overwhelmed. You'd be drowning in other people's noise.

The same thing happens in our heads.

Thought curation begins with awareness. When you notice a thought: maybe a worry, a memory, a flash of inspiration, you pause and ask:

• Is this helpful or harmful right now?
• Is this true, or just loud?
• Is this mine to carry, or something I picked up unconsciously?

These questions act like filters. They don't erase thoughts but they help you hold them with wisdom. Some thoughts are worth examining. Others are better off released.

This is where journaling, talking with trusted friends, or even sitting in quiet reflection can help; things we'll still discuss in full shortly. You begin to sort: *This idea energises me. This one shames me.* This one's not even mine; it's something I absorbed from social media. With time, you build an internal compass that knows what to keep, and what to gently lay down.

Science backs this up, too. A growing body of research around cognitive de-fusion; a practice within Acceptance and Commitment Therapy (ACT), teaches that we are not our thoughts. When we name them, step back, and choose how to relate to them, we reduce their power over us.

Mental Filing Systems: Organizing the Mind

Your mind is a brilliant processor and not a great storage unit. When we combine those deadlines, dreams, grocery lists, conversations we need to have, etc. in our heads, our mental space starts to feel like a desktop with 47 untitled files. You know everything's in there… somewhere but good luck finding it when you need it.

That's where mental filing systems come in.

By creating reliable, external structures to store and sort what matters, you reduce the pressure on your mind to remember everything. You give your brain permission to rest and focus on what it does best: thinking, not juggling.

Let's begin with the simplest and most powerful tools available: planners, lists, and frameworks.

Using Planners, Lists, and Frameworks

Our minds are not designed to carry everything at once. When we attempt to hold onto every task, appointment, idea, and worry in our heads, we create unnecessary strain. Mental clarity does not require doing more but it requires a reliable system that supports our thinking by organising it into manageable pieces.

This is where planners, lists, and frameworks become essential tools. When used intentionally, they function as external filing cabinets for the mind. They help you decide what matters, when it matters, and what can wait. Rather than depending on memory, you begin depending on structure. Let us explore each one in detail.

Planners: Creating Mental Boundaries Through Time

I've seen many people talk about planners but they don't actually get its use right. A planner is a boundary-setting tool for the mind. When you allocate time to a task or an event, you are giving your brain permission to stop holding onto it.

For example, if you need to follow up with a colleague about a report, writing it into your planner for Thursday at 11:00 a.m. tells your mind, "This has a place. You don't need to carry it right now."

This act of scheduling does two powerful things: it closes open loops and builds trust in your own system. You begin to believe that what needs to be done will be done because you've recorded it in a place you regularly return to. When I got to understand this, I began using planners and still use it to this very day.

Listen well: you need a planner!

Practical Activity:

• Choose one planning method that suits your life. It could be digital (such as Google Calendar or Notion) or paper-based (a weekly planner or agenda).

• Begin each week by blocking time for both essential tasks and personal anchors. Include rest, thinking time, and even ten-minute pauses.

• Each evening, review the next day's entries and prepare mentally. These routine grounds your sense of direction.

Lists: Lightening the Mental Load Through Categorisation

While planners handle when, lists handle what. They provide a direct, uncluttered way to move ideas and obligations out of your head and into a form you can interact with. Not every thought or task requires immediate action. However, until it is placed somewhere, your brain continues to cycle it. Lists allow you to clear that backlog.

From personal experience and conversations with others, I'd like you to know that there is no perfect list; only a useful one. Some people prefer categorised task lists. Others use simple running logs. The key is consistency and accessibility and that's all that should matter to you. Your list should be easy to update and hard to ignore.

Practical Activity:
- Create three distinct lists in a dedicated notebook or app:
   1. Today's Priorities: Limit this to three tasks that will move your day forward meaningfully.
   2. The Capture List: A running space for thoughts, reminders, ideas, and things you're not yet ready to act on.
   3. The Not-Now List: A safe holding zone for good ideas or commitments you've chosen to delay without guilt.
- Set a time each evening to review, update, and reprioritise. This keeps your system fluid and alive.

Frameworks: Thinking Better Through Repetition and Structure

Frameworks are mental models that guide how we make decisions and organise information. It is like an already established theory based on what others have felt or experienced. They offer shape to our thoughts, especially in moments of uncertainty or overwhelm.

Without a framework, we tend to approach each situation from scratch, using up cognitive energy and emotional bandwidth. With a framework, we reduce the burden of decision-making and focus instead on discernment and follow-through.

There are many frameworks to choose from. The best ones are simple, repeatable, and flexible enough to adapt to different areas of life.

Practical Activity:
- Try the following beginner-friendly frameworks this week:
* **The Eisenhower Matrix:** Divide your tasks into four categories: urgent and important, important but not urgent, urgent but not important, and neither urgent nor important. This clarifies what deserves your attention first.
* **The Rule of Three:** Choose three outcomes per day and three per week. These should reflect what will make the day or week feel successful and not just busy.

* **Bullet Journaling:** Use a notebook to log short-form entries: tasks, notes, reflections, and ideas.

Each of these tools cultivates intentional thinking. They help you slow down, process more deeply, and act with alignment rather than reaction.

Externalising Memory for Peace of Mind

The truth is, memory is fallible. It is not a filing cabinet, but more like a whiteboard that gets smudged as we move through the day. As science would say, the brain forgets roughly 97% of the things that happens in a day. That's how good our memory is at moving on – pun intended.

Anyway, the more you try to retain, the more likely you are to feel scattered, anxious, or mentally burdened even if you have done very little that day. Externalising memory is the act of taking what you are trying to hold internally and placing it into a trusted, physical or digital system. This might include notebooks, calendars, apps, sticky notes, visual boards, or even voice recordings. I call it "memory journaling."

When you externalise memory, you create what researchers in cognitive science call "**extended cognition.**" This concept suggests that tools like notebooks or digital reminders become literal extensions of the brain.

The peace that comes from knowing everything has a place is profound. It allows your mind to stop clinging to details and begin engaging with ideas. It shifts your energy from remembering to *reflecting.*

Practical Activity: Build a Simple Memory Extension System

1. Select Your Tools

Choose tools you are likely to use daily. This could include:

o   A pocket-sized notebook or journal

o   A notes app or task manager (such as Apple Notes, Notion, Todoist, or Google Keep) o A wall calendar or visual planner

2. Create a Capture Routine

Establish specific times in the day to offload what's in your head. Morning and evening work well for most people. During those moments, ask yourself:
o What am I trying to remember right now?
o Is there something I've thought about more than once today?
o What decisions or follow-ups are floating around in my mind?

3. Organise Lightly, Review Often

You do not need perfect organisation, but you do need consistency. Group similar types of information (e.g., errands, long-term ideas, project notes). At the end of each day or week, review your entries. Update what needs action. Delete what no longer matters.

4. Make it Visible

If you rely only on digital storage, consider placing visual reminders in your environment. A whiteboard in your office, a corkboard in your kitchen, or sticky notes on your mirror can serve as mental anchors - gentle prompts that reduce internal tension.

Creating a "Mental Inbox" and "Outbox"

Still as a means of detoxing the mind by externalizing memory, you could create for yourself a mental inbox and outbox. In the world of productivity and information flow, we're familiar with the idea of an inbox; a space where new inputs land before we process them. We receive emails, messages, tasks, and ideas, and we sort through them one by one. But most of us do not use this principle in our internal world. We allow every thought to come in and swirl around without direction or a place to go. Over time, this creates mental congestion.

Creating a mental inbox and outbox gives your thoughts a practical structure. It is a way of acknowledging that your mind, like any workspace, needs a flow; a place for incoming information, and a process for outgoing resolution. Without it, we risk operating in a loop of mental backlog: too many thoughts started, too few followed through.

The Mental Inbox: Capturing New Inputs

Your mental inbox is where raw, unfiltered input is placed. This can include:
- Ideas that randomly come to you during the day
- Tasks someone mentions in passing
- Emotional reactions you want to process later
- A book recommendation or quote you heard
- A question you're pondering but haven't explored

The key here is *non-judgmental capturing*. Do not filter or organise yet. This is the holding space. Just like you wouldn't respond to every email the second it arrives, you don't need to act on every thought immediately.

Practical Activity:

1.   Designate a space (physical or digital) for your inbox. This might be a notes app labelled "Mental Inbox," a journal section, or a voice note app.
2.   Throughout the day, when something new pops into your mind, capture it. Keep it brief and natural.
3.   Choose one consistent time each day (or every other day) to review the inbox and decide what each item needs: action, reflection, delegation, or deletion.

The Mental Outbox: Processing and Releasing

Your mental outbox is where decisions, resolutions, and follow-ups go. It's the part of the process that brings closure.

Examples might include:
- A decision made after days of mental weighing
- A message sent or task completed

- A journal entry that helped you work through something
- A conversation that helped resolve tension
- A final "let it go" moment like choosing to release a thought or worry

Using a mental outbox helps your brain feel progress. It tells your inner world: "This is no longer pending." For you, this sensation of closure will be deeply restorative and energising.

Practical Activity:
1.   Create a dedicated section in your notebook or app titled "Outbox" or "Done and Dusted."
2.   At the end of each day or week, reflect: What did I process or resolve? What loop did I close? What thought no longer needs space in my mind?
3.   Write it down. This small habit creates a sense of psychological momentum which is a proof that your mind is moving forward, not spinning in place.

The Role of Boundaries in Mental Clarity

Now, for everything we do in life, we must consider the recurring term known as "boundaries." I define boundaries as the answer to the question, "How far can this go?" When we want to achieve mental detox and clarity, we must consider protection as one of the major sectors. This protection involves preserving your attention, emotional energy, and decision-making power. In a world that constantly asks for more, clearer thinking often begins with intentional *limiting*.

So, imagine boundaries to be your guideposts and not necessarily a blockage. They define where your responsibility ends and where someone else's begins. They help you honour your values, your capacity, and your wellbeing.

Without boundaries, your mind becomes like an open city: anyone can enter, anything can demand attention, and every interruption from people around you feel urgent. Over time, this erodes your ability to concentrate, reflect, or even recognise your own needs.

In this section, we will explore boundaries as tools of clarity. When used well, they free your mind to function as it was meant to: spacious, steady, and focused.

How Saying "No" is a Mental Health Tool

When we were growing up, we were taught to say yes as a sign of kindness, flexibility, or teamwork. At least, yes was wired towards positivity. We learned that saying "no" was rude, confrontational, or selfish. But as we step into more intentional living, we must unlearn that belief because every yes is also a no to something else. Often, that "something else" is your peace, your energy, or your most important work.

I've gotten to understand "no" to be a declaration of focus. In fact, there is no greater way to cultivate space in your life than to say no to the extremities of the outside world.

When you say yes to too many commitments, your attention gets pulled in multiple directions. You begin carrying responsibilities that were never meant to be yours. And mentally, this creates background noise; the kind that drains you before the day even starts.

Saying no, on the other hand, is an act of self-leadership. It is a way of choosing what matters most and protecting it from erosion. It is important to note, though, that not all no's need to sound like "no." They can sound like:

- "I'm unable to take that on right now."
- "I appreciate the offer, but I need to pass."
- "That doesn't align with my focus at the moment."
- "Thanks for thinking of me. I'm prioritising rest this week."

These responses are firm, but respectful.

Practical Reflection:
1. Take a moment to list the areas in your life where you feel stretched or mentally cluttered because of a commitment you made out of obligation rather than alignment.

2. Ask yourself: *What would change if I allowed myself to say no more often?*

3. Write down three "no" responses you can use this week. Keep them simple and authentic to your tone.

Guarding Attention Like a Resource

If time is your most precious currency, attention is how you spend it.

As we've discussed earlier, our world is built around an attention economy. What you pay attention to; you start to care about. And what you care about begins to shape your thoughts, your emotions, and ultimately, your direction.

This is why protecting your attention is a matter of mental and emotional wellbeing, particularly mental in this case. When your attention is scattered, everything begins to feel urgent. You jump from task to task, thought to thought, never quite landing anywhere. Over time, this constant partial focus wears down your clarity. You might feel mentally tired but unable to point to what you've actually done. You've spent energy, but not on the things that nourish or move you forward.

That's why guarding your attention, for me, means choosing what enters your mental space with greater intention. It requires awareness and boundaries. You must begin treating your attention as if it were money in a limited account; like something to be budgeted wisely, not handed out on impulse.

Practical Strategies for Protecting Your Attention:

1. **Design Your Digital Environment Intentionally** (We'll get into more of this in the next chapter).

2. **Time Block for Deep Work**

Dedicate blocks of time, even 30 minutes, to uninterrupted, single-focus work. During that time, silence your phone, close unnecessary browser tabs, and give your full presence to the task. Deep work is where mental clarity is often rediscovered.

3.   Guard Your Mornings and Evenings

Begin your day with intention, not information. Delay checking email or social media for the first 30–60 minutes. Likewise, create a wind-down ritual at night that allows your mind to settle without being pulled into fresh stimuli.

4.   Name Your Distractions

Keep a notepad nearby. When a distracting thought arises ("I need to send that email"), write it down. This allows your brain to release it without acting on it immediately.

5.   Be Mindful of Conversations That Drain You

Not every conversation deserves equal access. Notice which interactions leave you mentally cluttered and which ones offer clarity or calm. Guard your relational energy accordingly.

The Art of Building a Mental Silence Zone

A mental silence zone is the deliberate presence of stillness; a space where your thoughts are not being pulled, provoked, or polluted. I consider it to be both a physical arena and a state of mind. To achieve mental silence, you must pause from consumption, decision-making, responding, and performing. In this space, the mind is allowed to soften its grip and the noise settles.

Creating mental silence zones in your day offer a buffer between moments which allows you to reset, reorient, and reconnect with what matters most. And don't forget; it often needs a physical setting to support it.

Designing a Physical Space for Mental Stillness

You do not need a perfectly decorated room or expensive equipment to create a mental silence zone. You simply need a space that signals to your brain: here, we rest, reflect, and release so you can consider setting aside any of such space as you carry out your physical declutter. Here are practical steps to equip a physical space for mental stillness:

1.	**Choose a Consistent Spot**

Pick a corner of your home, a chair by a window, a seat in your garden, or even a particular step on your porch. I loved selecting the area that gives you a view. For me, it's the waterfront just beyond the study room. What matters is consistency. Over time, your mind will associate that space with calm and clarity just as you associate a bed with sleep.

2.	**Keep It Uncluttered and Simple**

No, I cannot overemphasize the need to keep this space free of any form of physical clutters. This is not a productivity zone. Remove distractions, screens, and items that demand action and attention. Keep the space minimal. You can have a cushion, a blanket, a plant, a candle, a journal.

3.	**Add Elements That Anchor You**

Consider objects that signal peace or presence:
- A soft lamp or natural light
- A sound machine or silence-enhancing earplugs
- A grounding scent (lavender oil, a cup of tea, or fresh air)
- A tactile object to hold (a smooth stone, a rosary, a calming object)

4.	**Use This Space with Intention, Not Obligation**

Don't look at this as a productivity hack and force yourself to have to pull it up every day. Just visit this space when you feel overstimulated, unfocused, or emotionally stretched. Use it to sit quietly, breathe, journal, stretch gently, or simply be without input.

Creating Pockets of Silence Within Your Day

While a physical space is powerful, you can also build smaller, invisible mental silence zones throughout your routine. These are brief moments where you unplug from doing and return to being.

Here are ways to integrate them:
- **Transition Moments:** Before switching from one task to another, pause for 60 seconds. Breathe. Do nothing. Let one moment end before the next begins.

• **Silent Morning Minutes:** Begin your day with five minutes of intentional silence. No phone, no planning, no reading.

• **Digital Fast Breaks:** Once a day, take a 30-minute break with no screens, news, or social input.

• **End-of-Day Unwinding:** Before bed, sit in silence with a cup of something warm. No content, no stimulation.

The Reset: Micro-Moments That Help You Detox Daily

In this section, we'll explore three types of micro-resets you can build into your daily rhythm. Each one is practical, interactive, and designed to work with your real life, not around it.

1. 5-Minute Checkouts

A 5-minute checkout is a conscious pause at key transition points in your day either morning, midday, or evening. As I would tell my students, it's a form of check-in, so that you can check out. This helps our brains close open loops, process emotion, and reset for what's next.

Here's a simple 5-minute script you can try:

Minute	Prompt	What to Do
Minute 1	*"What's on my mind right now?"*	Close your eyes or lower your gaze. Say or write whatever thoughts surface. No judgment. Just notice.
Minute 2	*"What am I feeling in my body?"*	Do a quick scan from head to toe. Are you tense? Tired? Wired? Restless? Acknowledge it.
Minute 3	*"What do I need most right now?"*	This could be something physical (water, food), emotional (reassurance), or practical (clarity). Just name it.

| Minute 4 | *"What can I release?"* | Exhale. Let go of one lingering thought, even if temporarily. Whisper it: "I can let this go." |
| Minute 5 | *"What matters next?"* | Choose one focus point moving forward - not a full list. Just one anchor. Then gently re-enter your day. |

Practice Tip: Set a gentle alarm on your phone to remind you of your preferred reset time perhaps 11:30 a.m. and 5:00 p.m. Over time, this becomes a ritual your nervous system will begin to crave.

2. Nature Breaks and Stimulus Fasts

In a stimulus-saturated world, our nervous systems are constantly processing. Without release, this builds up into mental static. One of the fastest ways to detox from it is to step outside and of course, reconnect with nature. I've seen people get this notion quite twisted, thinking they literally need to be Mowgli to get this right. Nope, you don't need a forest. A balcony, a tree-lined street, or even standing by an open window works.

Let's try a Nature Reset Practice right now:

Step 1: Step away from your current space even if it's just a walk to the garden, front door, or nearest patch of daylight.

Step 2: Look outward. Pick one natural object like a leaf, a shadow, the sky, the movement of light. Gaze at it for one minute without naming or analysing it.

Step 3: Stay unplugged. No phone, no music, no camera.

Now, take note - how does your body feel after just three minutes? This is the power of a *stimulus* fast.

Stimulus fasts are short periods when you intentionally reduce input. Even 20 minutes of being in a quiet, natural environment without needing to produce or respond restores mental space.

Reset Option	Duration	Ideal Frequency
Nature break (light walk or gaze)	5–15 minutes	Once or twice a day
Window moment (no phone, no talking)	2 minutes	Every 2–3 hours
Full stimulus fast (no screens, no talking, no tasks)	20–30 minutes	Once every 2–3 days

3. Breathing and Body-Based Grounding Techniques

Your breath is your most accessible reset tool and your body is your fastest way back to presence. So, you don't mess with it. When your mind is racing or scattered, trying to "think your way into calm" rarely works. But dropping into the body allows calm to arise from the inside out. These grounding techniques can be used in private or public, standing or sitting. They are quiet, portable, and powerful.

Let's walk through a **Simple Grounding Reset** you can practice anywhere.

The 3–3–3 Breath
- Inhale for 3 counts
- Hold for 3 counts
- Exhale for 3 counts
- Repeat 3 times

This slows the heart rate, resets the nervous system, and grounds the mind.
Now pair it with a physical anchor:

The 3–2–1 Body Anchor
- Name 3 things you can feel physically (e.g., your feet on the floor, your hands on your lap, your back against the chair)

- Name 2 things you can hear
- Name 1 thing you can smell or taste

Together, these pull your attention gently back into the present. To help keep these resets alive, consider printing or saving a visual tracker like this:

Day	5-Minute Checkout	Nature Break / Stimulus Fast	Breath or Body Grounding
Monday	□ Morning □ Evening	□ Window □ Walk	□ Breathwork
Tuesday	□ Morning □ Evening	□ Window □ Walk	□ Breathwork
Wednesday	...	...	...

Use simple ticks or notes to mark the days you practice.
These micro-moments are small enough to fit into any day, yet powerful enough to transform your mental landscape over time.

The Weekly Reset: Staying Mentally Clear Long-Term

The real art isn't decluttering once - it's staying clear even as life keeps coming.

You know how people do a huge closet clean-out and swear they'll never let it get that bad again, then six months later they're right back to "I have nothing to wear"? Mental clarity can be the same.

The trick isn't a once-and-for-all brain detox but building tiny systems that keep you clear, as life happens. Let's explore three powerful, sustainable practices that help you stay mentally clear over the long haul.

1. Weekly Check-ins and Mental Audits

I like to think of this like brushing your mental teeth. You wouldn't skip brushing for a week and expect to feel fresh. In the same way, a weekly check-in clears the small buildup before it becomes a mental cavity.

Let me tell you about a friend of mine, Suzan. She's a project manager, mum of three... I suggested a weekly mental audit; nothing complicated, just 20 minutes every Sunday evening to review the week and reset for the next. Within a month, she said these and it stuck with me, *"I didn't know how much tension I was carrying until I started letting it go."*

Try This: Your Weekly Mental Check-in

Set aside 20–30 minutes once a week (Sunday night or Monday morning works well). Use these four prompts:

Prompt	What to Reflect On
What drained me this past week?	Identify situations, people, or habits that felt heavy.
What gave me clarity or joy?	Highlight moments of peace, alignment, or energy.
What's unfinished that I'm still mentally carrying?	Make a list. Decide what to schedule, delegate, or release.
What do I want next week to feel like?	Focus on a desired mental state, not just a to-do list.

Optional Tip: Keep a dedicated *Mental Check-In* Notebook. You'll start noticing patterns: what regularly clutters your mind, and what regularly clears it.

2. Habit Stacking for Clarity

Have you ever brushed your teeth without realising it? Or brewed your coffee on autopilot? That's the magic of habit and when used intentionally, it becomes a powerful clarity tool.

Habit stacking means attaching a new mental health habit to an existing routine. You don't add pressure or carve out new time but simply layer clarity into what you're already doing.

Let me paint you a picture.

Try This: Your Habit Stack Builder

Use the table below to build your own stack:

Current Habit	New Mental Clarity Add-On	What It Supports
Brushing teeth	Breathe deeply 3 times while looking in the mirror	Grounding before the day begins
Boiling water / waiting for kettle	Journal 3 lines: How am I feeling?	Emotional check-in
Walking the dog	Mentally repeat a mantra: "I release what I can't control."	Mental detox
Turning off computer	Write 1 thing I'm grateful for in a sticky note	Perspective shift

3. Designing a "Mental Maintenance" Routine

Just like your car needs regular servicing, your mind benefits from ongoing care. Not just emergency support when things feel chaotic but small rituals that keep things running smoothly.

Here's how I created my routine and you can do the same.

My Routine Snapshot (A Real-Life Example):

Daily (10 mins)	Weekly (30 mins)	Monthly (1 hour)
3-minute morning journal: "What matters today?" Silent tea or coffee, no phone	Sunday night review: brain dump, plan top 3 goals, reflect on week	End-of-month reflection: revisit journal entries, identify patterns, release unfinished things
Breath check before bed	Nature walk without phone	Schedule an "unplugged day" - offline, quiet, reflective

This routine isn't rigid. Some weeks I miss a day, or the nature walk becomes a 5-minute window stare. That's okay. What matters is the rhythm, not the ritual.

Design Your Own Mental Maintenance Routine

Complete this exercise:

1. **Choose a daily anchor.** What's one thing you can do for 5–10 minutes that brings your mind peace?

2. **Pick a weekly ritual.** What time works best to pause, reset, and reflect without rush?

3. **Schedule a monthly clean-out.** Book time now to do a deeper mental review. Celebrate what you're learning about yourself. Write it out. Name it. Post it somewhere visible.

Tools & Prompts for the Journey

As I wrap up this chapter, I'd want you to understand that this journey will look different for everyone. Some days you'll feel focused and grounded. Other days, you'll be knee-deep in mental mess wondering where your thoughts went. That's normal.

What makes the difference is having tools. They are simple, flexible anchors that pull you back into focus, perspective, and peace when the fog sets in and that's why I'd sum this up with the many self-made tools that I crafted overtime from my own meditative experiences.

Below are practical tools and prompts you can use again and again. Adapt them. Print them. Save them in your notes app. Revisit them whenever you need to re-centre.

1. Brain Dump Prompts

When your mind feels full, scattered, or overloaded - these help you get it out and clear the internal clutter.

Try this: Open a blank page and write freely for 5–10 minutes using one or more of the prompts below.

Prompt	What It Unlocks
"Right now, my brain feels like..."	Identifies emotional tone
"What I can't stop thinking about is..."	Surfaces mental clutter
"Here's everything I feel behind on..."	Eases pressure through listing
"If I had one hour of calm, I would..."	Reconnects with priorities
"What I wish I could say is..."	Releases unspoken thoughts

Pro Tip: After the dump, highlight one thing to act on and one thing to let go of. Small steps forward. Big mental relief.

2. Weekly Planning Template

A gentle, flexible planner that focuses less on tasks and more on mental direction.

Section	What to Write
Top 3 Priorities	What actually matters this week?

Emotional Focus	How do I want to feel by Friday? (e.g., steady, light, focused)
Unfinished Business	Anything from last week I'm still mentally carrying?
Space for Self	What is one thing I'll do just for me?
Boundaries to Set	Where do I need to say "no" or pause to protect clarity?
Encouragement Note	A mantra or reminder to guide me (e.g., "I don't have to do it all to be enough.")

Optional Tip: Fill this out every Sunday evening or Monday morning. It turns chaos into clarity before the week even begins.

3. Mental Noise Tracker

This is a tool to help you notice the pattern of your mental clutter like what's recurring, what's triggering, and what needs addressing rather than avoiding.

Date	What's Cluttering My Mind?	Theme	Next Step or Note
July 23	That email I haven't replied to	Avoidance	Schedule it for Thursday
July 23	Comparing myself to a friend	Insecurity	Journal about what's mine
July 24	Feeling like I'm always behind	Overcommitment	Revisit task list, trim it

Use this for one week. You'll start to see what thoughts keep coming back - those are the ones asking to be understood, not just managed.

4. Go-To Grounding Practices List

Make a personalised list of activities that help you reset quickly; just short, accessible re-centres.

Length of Time	Reset Options
1 minute	3 deep breaths with eyes closed
3 minutes	Step outside and look at the sky
5 minutes	Slow stretch and drink water mindfully
10 minutes	Write "what I feel and why" in a journal
20+ minutes	Take a walk, no phone - just you and your thoughts

Print it. Post it. When your brain feels like it's spinning, glance at the list and choose what's possible now.

5. Final Prompts for Deeper Clarity

These are reflective prompts for when you feel lost, stuck, or overwhelmed. Use them monthly or whenever you need a deeper reset.

- What has felt noisy lately - and what do I need to quiet?
- Which areas of my life feel heavy - and which feel light?
- What have I been tolerating that no longer serves me?
- Who or what brings clarity into my life?
- If I gave myself full permission to reset, what would I change first?

Chapter Seven
Swipe Less, Live More: Taking Back Your Tech

It started with the flicker of a screen.

11:17 p.m.

You pick up your phone to check the time. That's it. Just the time. But there it is; a single notification, then five. A friend posted a story. A work email came in. A headline pings.

You tap. Scroll. Swipe. Blink.

Now it's 12:42 a.m. You're not even sure what you were looking for anymore. In this chapter, we'll be taking back our power of our digital life and space together and it won't be by cutting tech out... Oh, no! Not when the world is now wired towards the digital space and not being inclined towards some digital platform is like being an ape-man among the civilized. What we'll be doing is cutting it all down to size because when your devices serve you - and not the other way around - you finally get to show up for the life that's been waiting on the other side of the screen.

Assess Your Digital Landscape

Before you declutter, you need to see the whole mess. You wouldn't start cleaning your house without walking through each room first, right? Same goes for your digital life. You can't declutter what you haven't consciously identified. Most of us are overwhelmed not because we have too much tech but because we've never taken time to actually map it out.

So yes, when I began the journey towards a seamless digital life, I took the first step of actually comprehending how much tech I had within my space. This is the part no one teaches us: how to audit the digital life we've built, app by app, platform by platform, file by file, until we see it clearly because once you see the full picture, everything else gets easier.

This next activity is designed to help you surface it all: your devices, subscriptions, tools, platforms, social media accounts, digital storage, screen habits, notifications, and more. Take your time here. This is the digital equivalent of opening every drawer.

Activity: The Full-Spectrum Digital Inventory

A 360° *walk through your digital ecosystem*

You can do this in a notebook, a spreadsheet, a journaling app, or by printing the following table. The goal is to map and not fix (yet). That comes next. Use the tables I've given below as guides to craft yours.

Step 1: Device Inventory - What's in Your Digital Hands?

Device	Purpose (Primary Use)	Hours Used Daily	Last Software Update	Notes
Phone	e.g., Messaging, Social, Work	5 hrs	March 2024	Too many apps
Laptop	Work, Writing	6 hrs	April 2024	Desktop cluttered
Tablet	Media consumption	3 hrs	February 2024	Mostly passive use
Smart-watch	Fitness tracking	Daily	Auto-updates	Notifications distracting
Other (TVs, Consoles, etc.)	Gaming, Streaming	2 hrs	-	Used late at night

Reflection Prompt:
- Which device do I instinctively reach for when I'm bored, anxious, or tired?
- Which one actually adds value and which one just drains me?

Step 2: App & Platform Inventory - What Lives on Your Devices?

Make four columns on a blank page or spreadsheet.

Category	Apps & Platforms	Frequency of Use	Energy Impact (− / + / 0)
Social Media	Instagram, Facebook, X	5–10x/day	− (comparison), 0 (passive)
Messaging	WhatsApp, Slack, Email	Constantly	+ (connection), − (interruptions)
Productive	Notion, Google Docs	3x/day	+ (work & planning)
Passive/Entertainment	YouTube, Netflix, Reddit	Evening use	− (time suck), + (relaxation)

Reflection Prompt:
- Which apps help me create or connect?
- Which ones do I scroll without remembering what I saw?

Step 3: Storage & File Ecosystem - What's Hiding in the Cloud?

This includes your digital "closets": file folders, drives, cloud accounts, downloads, and media.

Storage Zone	Type of Content	Organisation Level (1–10)	Clutter Score (Low / Medium / High)	Action Needed
Google Drive	Work, PDFs	3	High	Purge folders

Desktop	Screen-shots, Docs	4	Medium	Organise by project
Downloads	Random files	2	High	Mass delete
iCloud/ Photos	7,000+ photos	6	Medium– High	Archive/de-lete
External Drive	Old back-ups	7	Low	Possibly archive

Reflection Prompt:
- Where do I lose time searching for files?
- What needs archiving, deleting, or backing up?

Step 4: Subscriptions, Accounts & Logins - What's Running in the Background?

Service	Use Case	Monthly Cost	Logged In? (Y/N)	Keep / Cancel / Reassess
Spotify	Music	£9.99	Yes	Keep
Canva Pro	Design	£10.99	Yes	Reassess (use less now)
Audible	Audio-books	£7.99	Yes	Cancel
Amazon Prime	Delivery/ Media	£8.99	Yes	Keep

Reflection Prompt:
- Are these services serving me or are they cluttering my wallet and attention?

Step 5: Notifications, Inputs & Alerts - What's Trying to Get My Attention?

Device	Notifications On	Most Frequent Alerts	Helpful or Distracting?	Turn Off? (Y/N)
Phone	Yes	WhatsApp, Instagram, News	Mostly distracting	Yes
Laptop	Slack, Email	Work-related	Helpful during work hrs	No (set DND)

Reflection Prompt:

- How often am I interrupted while trying to focus?
- What would happen if I missed nothing for two hours?

Final Reflection: What's the State of My Digital Landscape?

Now that you've walked through your digital "home," ask:

- Where does most of my digital clutter live - in apps? files? alerts? time spent?
- Which three areas drain me the most?
- Which two tools or systems are actually helping me feel clearer?

Tame Your Device & App Chaos

Imagine unlocking your phone and seeing only what you actually use, what genuinely serves you, and what sparks something useful or joyful. The thing about the digital space clutter is that we didn't plan to have it all stuffed up. Apps accumulated one download at a time either for work, workouts, friends, hobbies, emergencies, trends, and things we forgot we even signed up for. However, currently, your screen feels noisy, your folders are unrecognisable and every time you open your phone, your mind loses just a little more focus.

Let's fix that.

The App Chaos Reset: A Flowchart Walk-through

Use this as a mental visual guide or sketch it on paper as you go.

Start Here: Your Home Screen

1. Open your phone

2. Take a deep breath

3. Ask: Does this screen reflect who I am now - or who I used to be online?

Now move through the chart below (mentally or literally) with each app.

```
                [Is this app still relevant to my life?]

                          |

              Yes ------------------ No

               |                 |

        [Do I use it weekly or more?]   --> Uninstall it

               |

           Yes ----------------- No

           |            |

  [Is it useful, joyful or creative?]   --> Archive it or move off home
  screen

               |

         Yes --------- No

           |      |

        Keep it    Move to folder labelled "Reassess Later"

               |
```

[Group it by function: Social, Work, Tools, Creativity]

The 15-Minute App Audit Challenge

Set a timer for 15 minutes. Pick one screen or one folder at a time. Here's how you spend those 15 minutes:

- **Minute 1–2:** Quick scan of your home screen. Identify the apps you've forgotten about.

- **Minute 3–10:** Apply the flowchart above. Delete, move, archive. Be decisive.

- **Minute 11–15:** Reorganise remaining apps by purpose and not by colour or brand, but function.

Recommended App Folder Labels:

- **Create:** Notes, Design, Writing, Music, Drawing
- **Connect:** Social media, Messaging, Email
- **Move:** Fitness, Health, Maps
- **Think:** Planning, Journals, Meditation
- **Tools:** Banking, Utilities, Passwords
- **Noise:** This is your "Maybe" folder - apps that feel like clutter but you're not ready to delete yet

Just like a clean kitchen invites better cooking, a clear phone invites better focus, creativity, and peace. One reader I worked with, James, was shocked to discover he had **143 apps** on his phone - but regularly used only 17. After the audit, he said, "I didn't realise how anxious my home screen was making me until I cleaned it. Now, opening my phone feels like a choice - not a trap."

Once you've finished, take a screenshot of your new home screen. Look at it. Breathe.

Does it feel lighter? More focused? More you?

Clean Up Your Files & Folders

You know that feeling when you clean out an old drawer and find a birthday card from 2018, 14 spare buttons, and three receipts you thought you needed?

That's what most of our laptops, cloud drives, and desktops have become. I call them "digital junk drawers."

The thing is mental load increases every time you stare at a cluttered screen especially for workers when you're trying to create, submit, or find something under pressure. We've all been here a couple of times either through school, or just a job. You waste minutes (sometimes hours) searching for that one PDF or sifting through 35 versions of "FINAL_v2_REALLYFINAL_USETHISONE.docx."

Let's clear that out.

Let's Begin: Here's What We Want to Achieve

You open your laptop and your desktop background is clear. There are no scattered files. Your folders are labelled and simple. You click "Documents" and know exactly where everything lives. No duplicates.

That's what we're building now.

The Folder Framework: Your Mega-System Simplified

Before you can clean, you need a system that can hold what matters and hide what doesn't. take a pause and read that again. Here's a no-fuss, four-folder system that works across computers, cloud storage, and even phones.

The 4 Mega-Folders:

1. **Work** - Projects, documents, presentations, proposals, resumes

2. **Personal** - Journals, ID scans, personal documents, forms

3. **Media** - Photos, videos, graphics, audio, social content

4. **Money & Admin** - Invoices, bank statements, tax forms, receipts

Everything you own fits somewhere in here.

Now Try This:

- Create these four folders on your desktop or cloud storage
- Drag all your scattered files into a temporary folder titled "SORT ME"
- Each day, spend 10–15 minutes moving files from **"SORT ME"** into the right mega-folder
- If you're not sure what something is, open it or toss it
- Don't overthink the process

The File Purge Sprint: 20-Minute Game On

Set a timer for 20 minutes. Play your favourite music. And tackle one of these zones:

- Your Downloads Folder
- Your Desktop
- Google Drive or iCloud
- Photo Gallery
- WhatsApp/Telegram Media Folders

Here's the goal you should have in mind: Delete duplicates, junk, and things you haven't opened in 6+ months.

Ask yourself:

- Have I used this in the past year?
- Do I have this saved somewhere else already?
- Will I ever need this again?

If not, let it go. Don't become the digital equivalent of a storage unit commercial.

Grace, a remote worker, once told me she spent 90 minutes looking for her passport scan while trying to book an urgent visa appointment. "I had six different folders, and no idea which laptop I'd saved it on. I literally cried in front of the embassy page." After implementing the mega-folder system, she messaged me months later: "I can find anything in under 30 seconds. I even made a folder called 'Important Adulting Things.' My brain thanks me daily." Your brain can thank you too!

Bonus Pro Tip: Archive, Don't Hoard

Create an "_ARCHIVE" folder inside each mega-folder. That's where old versions, expired documents, or former projects go to sleep.

It's not deleted and it's just not shouting at you anymore.

Inbox Zero & Email Management

There's a quiet kind of overwhelm that comes from opening your inbox every day and seeing the number "3,174" staring back at you like a digital accusation. I had over 20,000. I'm sure there are people with much higher numbers, especially those who keep multiple email accounts.

Let me tell you how this all came about. The problem is that email, for most people, stopped being a communication tool and started becoming a cluttered junk drawer of newsletters you didn't ask for, tasks you forgot to track, and digital receipts for things you don't even remember buying.

Let's be honest. Nobody taught us how to manage email. We were handed an address, and then, slowly but surely, it spiralled into this weird hybrid of to-do list, social feed, storage unit, and existential dread. But here's the good news. You don't need to reply to every message. You just need to get your inbox to a place that no longer weighs on your mind every time you open it.

Let's start with the easiest win: **get rid of the noise**. I'm talking about those promotional emails from brands you never bought from, the newsletters you signed up for during a midnight productivity high, or alerts from "online tools" you stopped using three careers ago.

You don't need to go through them one by one. Just search by sender or keyword and batch delete. It'll take less time than you think, and you won't miss them. Trust me. The peace of seeing an empty promotions tab? Underrated bliss.

Now comes the satisfying part: **clearing your main inbox**. You have two options here. There's the slow, careful clean-up or the bold reset. If your inbox is under 500 unread emails, you might choose the careful route. Scroll, delete, archive, repeat. But if you're staring at anything over 1,000? It's time for a bulk archive. Create a folder called "Inbox Freeze" and move everything into it. Yes, everything. Why? Because most of those emails are outdated, irrelevant, or will never be read anyway. And anything truly important will find its way back to you.

From this fresh start, you can now build a system that works with your brain. **Use folders or labels sparingly**. Not 50 micro-categories. Just a few broad ones like "Action," "Waiting," and "Reference." That way, when a new email comes in, you have a place to tuck it away if you're not dealing with it immediately.

And speaking of immediate, bring in the 2-minute rule. If the email takes less than two minutes to handle, do it now. Reply, forward, delete, file - whatever needs to happen. If it takes longer, drag it to your "Action" folder or flag it. This small shift alone will prevent that dreaded scroll of emails you meant to reply to but lost track of somewhere between Monday and "how is it already Friday?"

Now let's talk **boundaries**. Email isn't just about clutter but also access. You train your inbox the same way you train people: by how and when you respond. You don't owe anyone 24/7 access to your attention so try setting a time block. Maybe 30 minutes in the morning and 30 minutes in the late afternoon. Outside of that, your inbox can wait. The world will keep turning.

And don't underestimate the power of **unsubscribing**. It's like decluttering your digital mailbox at the root. Use tools like Clean Email, Unroll.me, or just the trusty "unsubscribe" link buried at the bottom of the newsletter. It's small, but deeply liberating. It's like quietly quitting from the noise.

Lastly, **celebrate your progress**. Even if you don't hit zero right away, notice how much lighter you feel.

Inbox Reset Checklist

Use this checklist to put everything above into motion. It's designed to be simple, empowering, and repeatable. You can print it, save it to your notes app, or check things off in real time.

Clear the Junk

- ☐ Open the "Promotions" or "Social" tab
- ☐ Search for known brands you no longer engage with
- ☐ Batch delete 50 or more irrelevant messages
- ☐ Unsubscribe from 3 or more newsletters

Archive the Past

- ☐ Create a new folder named "Inbox Freeze"
- ☐ Select all messages older than 30 days
- ☐ Move them to "Inbox Freeze"

Organise the Present

- ☐ Create 3 folders: "Action," "Waiting," "Reference"
- ☐ Move current tasks into "Action"
- ☐ Move messages pending responses into "Waiting"
- ☐ Store receipts, documents, etc. in "Reference"

Apply the 2-Minute Rule

- ☐ Skim the most recent 10–15 emails
- ☐ Handle what you can in under 2 minutes
- ☐ Flag or file the rest into "Action"

Set Your Boundaries

- ☐ Choose two time blocks per day for checking email
- ☐ Turn off push notifications
- ☐ Add a "response hours" note to your signature (optional)

Celebrate Small Wins

☐ Give yourself something: a tea break, a walk, a playlist

Digital Input Audit & Content Curation

Let's get honest. Your phone is more than just some tool but also a portal to information that can make or mar you as we've discussed in earlier chapters. Every scroll, swipe, or "suggested for you" moment is feeding your brain something and as it is with any diet, what you consume regularly will begin to shape how you think, how you feel, and who you believe you are.

This section is here to help you choose because your content diet is a lot like your food diet: if you're constantly snacking on mental junk, you'll stay mentally bloated. But with just a few intentional shifts, you can create a feed that fuels clarity, focus, and even joy.

Build Your Digital Menu

Grab a notebook, notes app, or open a fresh page in your journal. You're about to craft your very own Digital Menu; a curated guide to what's allowed into your mental ecosystem.

Step 1: Audit Your Current Feed

Answer these quick, honest prompts:

Morning Feed:

What's the first thing I usually consume online each morning?

Does it make me feel grounded or agitated?

Scroll Mood:

What mood am I usually in when I start scrolling?

What mood am I in after?

Most Visited Apps (Last 3 Days):

Check your phone settings. Which apps or websites are eating your screen time?

Types of Content I Consume Most:

Inspirational, educational, news, gossip, memes, productivity tips, comparison-driven influencers, niche hobbies?

Who do I follow that regularly lifts me up?

Who do I follow out of habit, guilt, or boredom?

Write freely.

Step 2: Categorise Your Feeds (Using the "Pantry Method")

Imagine your digital life like a kitchen pantry. Use the categories below to mentally sort your content:

Category	What Goes Here
Nourishing	Content that inspires, educates, or soothes. These are your digital veggies.
Neutral	Content you enjoy casually but doesn't impact your mood either way.
Numbing	Content you consume out of habit, escape, or to avoid something else.
Noisy	Content that drains you, triggers anxiety, or encourages comparison.

Take a look at your recent follows, subscriptions, and go-to platforms. Place them into these buckets. You might be surprised.

Step 3: Curate Your Digital Menu

Now it's time to design your intentional intake. Use the builder below to guide your choices.

Platforms I Intend to Keep Using:

(e.g. Instagram, YouTube, Pinterest, Twitter/X)

→ Why are they staying?

→ What boundaries or time limits will I set for them?

Accounts I Want to Follow More Of:

(e.g. Creators who teach, uplift, or help me think deeply)

→ List 3 people or pages to seek out this week.

Content I'm Detoxing From:

→ Unfollow 3 creators or mute 3 topics that no longer serve you.

→ Bonus: Unsubscribe from 3 YouTube channels or newsletters you never open.

Digital Meal Prep (New Habits):

→ Instead of scrolling in bed, I'll...

→ Before I open social media, I'll check in with how I feel.

→ I'll schedule "screen snacks" instead of grazing all day long.

Optional Weekly Ritual: The 15-Minute Content Cleanse

Once a week, take 15 minutes to:

• Unfollow or mute accounts that drained you

• Revisit saved posts you haven't looked at

• Archive old podcasts, subscriptions, or email lists

• Refill your feed with things that reflect who you're becoming, not just who you've been

Notification & Attention Management

There's this moment that happens to the best of us: you're halfway through a thought, finally focused on something meaningful, and then - ding. Your phone lights up. Group chat... Another one... App update... Calendar alert... Suddenly, the thought is gone, like steam vanishing from a mirror.

And just like that, your attention is hijacked. Most times, when we try to go back to those thoughts, we realize they are actually gone! Especially if they were creative in nature.

Notifications are designed to be irresistible. We see bright bubbles, haptic taps, colours that scream "urgent" when the thing being delivered is anything but that.

The truth is, you can't stay focused if your brain is trained to flinch every 45 seconds. And you can't feel peaceful if your devices are constantly throwing things at you. Somewhere along the line, we accepted that everything needed our attention now. But that's a myth. And we're done with it.

Let's start simple. Your phone does not need to notify you every time something happens inside it. It's not a toddler needing constant supervision. You're allowed to **mute it**. You're allowed to choose what's worth your focus and what can wait.

Start by going through your notifications the same way you'd clean out your wardrobe. Ask: *Does this serve me, or is it just making noise?* That notification from the food delivery app telling you it's burger night? Gone. The 6:00 a.m. news update that kicks off your cortisol levels before your feet hit the floor? Definitely gone. You don't have to cut it all off, but you do get to **curate**.

For apps you use regularly like messages, email, or calendars, try switching them to **badge-only or scheduled delivery**. You'll still see what matters, but your phone won't be acting like it's trying to win an attention Olympics every hour. For everything else? Turn it off. No really, off.

And then there's **Do Not Disturb mode**. If you're not using it, you're missing one of the best mental health tools already built into your phone. Schedule it. Use it while you work. Use it while you eat. Use it while you think. The world won't crumble because you didn't check your WhatsApp in the past seven minutes.

You can even go a step further. Try setting your screen to **grayscale** when you're deep in work. It's less stimulating, less addictive, and somehow makes scrolling lose its flavour kind of like eating crisps without salt. It is surprisingly effective.

Now, let's talk home screen real estate. If your first page is full of noise from social media apps, breaking news, or red-dot drama and the likes, try relocating those apps. Hide them in folders or move them to the second or third screen. This tiny act adds friction, which gives your brain a chance to ask: *Do I really want to open this, or am I just reaching out of habit?*

Finally, you get to build a quieter phone.

Passwords, Privacy & Device Health

Welcome to your not-so-annual digital check-up. Don't worry, no one's judging you for using the same password since 2014 or ignoring that "Update Available" notification for three weeks straight. We've all been there.

But here's the deal. Your devices whether phone, laptop, tablet, smartwatch, maybe even your fridge, are the digital equivalent of organs in today's life. If they're bloated or infected, it affects you more than you think.

So let's put on the metaphorical white coat and do a full-body scan of your digital health.

SECTION A: Passwords - Let's Talk About Those Keys

Patient Status:

Be honest. Are your passwords:

A) All the same with a number at the end

B) Stored in your head and three different notebooks

C) Saved in your browser because you forgot them all

D) Managed by a secure password manager

If you answered A through C, congratulations - you're completely normal. And also extremely vulnerable.

What to Do Next:

Start using a password manager. I'm not talking about your browser (though the autofill browser features work just fine), or your dog's name, but an actual encrypted tool like **Bitwarden, 1Password,** or Dashlane. They generate strong passwords, remember them for you, and sync across devices. You only need to remember one master password and not 37 variations of "Butterfly2020!"

Choose your top 5 most sensitive accounts (banking, email, cloud storage, social media, work tools) and change those passwords first. The rest can follow gradually.

Also: enable **two-factor authentication (2FA)** anywhere it's offered. It's the digital equivalent of locking your front door and setting the alarm. One more step for you, a thousand steps for anyone trying to break in.

SECTION B: Privacy - Who's Watching You Scroll?

Patient Status:

Do you know which apps have access to your camera, location, microphone, or contacts?

No? That's okay. Neither do most people.

Some of your apps are collecting far more than they need. And while you're living your best life, they're quietly building little data profiles like a nosy neighbour with a spreadsheet.

What to Do Next:

Visit your device's privacy settings. Go through permissions like you're Marie Kondo-ing your digital closet.

Ask: *Does this flashlight app really need my exact location?*

No? Revoke access.

Do a full sweep of your app permissions. Turn off unnecessary access to your microphone, photos, and contacts. Then check which third-party platforms are connected to your Google or Facebook accounts. Revoke any you no longer use. Trust me - you will not miss that quiz app from 2017.

SECTION C: Device Health - Time for a Digital Detox Bath

Patient Status:

How often do you restart your devices, run updates, or scan for viruses?

A) Rarely

B) Only when something breaks

C) Updates make me nervous

D) I love a clean OS and fresh cache

If you're not at D yet, you're in good company. But here's the catch: things might look fine until they're not.

What to Do Next:

- Run all pending software updates across your devices
- Update your apps (yes, even the ones you haven't opened in months)
- Restart your phone and laptop at least once a week
- Run a malware scan (use Malwarebytes, Avast, or built-in tools like Windows Defender or Apple's Gatekeeper)

Think of this as the digital equivalent of clearing out your sinuses. Less clutter, fewer bugs, and everything runs smoother.

Doctor's Notes & Encouragement

You are allowed to be someone who loves tech and refuses to be careless with it. You are allowed to be someone who streams, scrolls, works, and creates without giving away every piece of your identity to the algorithm gods. So this is your reminder. Update. Protect. Clean out the cobwebs. Your future self will thank you. And your phone might finally stop overheating while doing absolutely nothing.

Plan a Digital Detox or Sabbath

Now, let's carry out a digital exorcism. Before you freak out, it's not exactly how it seems. Alright, let's just call it a pause. *Phew.*

Irrespective, that's where a detox or digital sabbath comes in. A digital detox is a break that gives people the permission to be unavailable, to go quiet or to basically carry out a break without still capturing it on your stories. So, nope... you don't need to update those TikTok or Insta fans just how well it's going. I've always hated that fake attention.

Below, you'll create your own custom detox, choosing the flavour, duration, and vibe that fits your life right now.

Choose Your Detox Type

    1.   The Espresso Shot (2–6 hours)

Perfect for a focused morning, a long walk, or dinner with someone you love. No phone, no laptop, no notifications. Just presence.

    2.   The Half-Day Reset (6–12 hours)

Ideal for a slow weekend, a deep creative work session, or a full afternoon in nature. You're reachable only if it's urgent - and not through Instagram.

    3.   The Full-Day Sabbath (24 hours)

This is the classic. One full day offline. No social, no email, no "just checking." Think books, board games, bike rides. Bonus points for naps.

    4.   The Full Cleanse (72 hours+)

More ambitious, but wildly freeing. Great for travel, retreats, birthdays, or emotional reboots. You'll be amazed how fast your brain remembers it was designed to be still.

Build Your Detox Plan

Use this section like a custom planner. Circle your choices or journal your responses.

Start Date & Time:

When will it begin? Be specific. This creates accountability.

End Time (or soft finish):

When will you check back in? Decide before you start - it keeps the loop clean.

Devices on Pause:

Phone

Laptop

Tablet

TV

Smartwatch

Other: _____

Allowed Tech (if any):

Maybe you'll use your Kindle or you'll play vinyl. Or let's go it's strictly analogue. You decide.

Who Needs to Know I'm Offline?

Let key people know ahead of time. A simple "Hey, taking a digital reset, I'll be back [insert time]" message does the trick.

Backup Plan for Emergencies:

Who can reach you and how? Have one line open or pass messages through someone if needed.

Replacement Activities Menu

With the space we've created together, there'll be vacuums. Let's fill those up. Choose 5+ from this list or add your own:

• Read a book with actual pages

• Take a slow walk and name what you see

• Bake something from scratch

• Sketch, doodle, or journal

• Deep clean a room (yes, this counts)

• Sit in silence and sip something warm

• Visit a local spot you've ignored

• Write a letter - like with a pen

• Nap with zero guilt

• Play board games, build a puzzle, or learn a card trick

• Do absolutely nothing on purpose

When You Return

Take 10 minutes to reflect before you open any apps. Ask:

•   What did I miss that actually mattered?

- What didn't I miss at all?
- What do I want to change going forward?

This is the real gift of the detox. It doesn't just clear time but also clears perspective.

Keep It Clear: Maintenance & Habit Design

So, you've cleaned up your digital chaos. Your inbox is lighter. Your apps are under control. Notifications no longer rule your mood. And for the first time in a long time, your devices feel like tools again and not tiny tyrants in your pocket.

Now the question is: how do you *keep* it that way?

Digital clutter, like physical clutter, has a sneaky way of creeping back in. You need maintenance that feels more like *self-respect* than self-discipline.

The Weekly "Clean Sweep"

Once a week - maybe on a Sunday evening or during your quiet Monday coffee - take 15 to 20 minutes to reset your digital space:

- Delete screenshots, downloads, and random photos that no longer serve you
- Close all browser tabs you forgot you opened
- Tidy up your desktop or phone home screen
- Review your calendar and delete outdated reminders
- Check your email folders for lingering clutter and archive what's done

This mini-routine keeps the dust from building up.

The Monthly File Audit

Once a month, pick a date (like the first Saturday) and do a deeper dive:

- Organize your folders (Work, Personal, Media, Finance, etc.)
- Move completed projects into archives

- Back up your files to the cloud or an external drive
- Run software updates on all devices
- Delete any unused apps that have crept back in

Pro tip: set a recurring calendar event for this. Make it sacred. Pour a drink, put on music, and make it feel like a spa day for your files.

"One In, One Out" Rule

This is digital minimalism made simple. Every time you install a new app, subscribe to a new email list, or start using a new tool, pause and ask:

What can I let go of in exchange?

Maybe it's a podcast you no longer enjoy, an app you haven't opened in two months, or a subscription that no longer adds value. Trade as you go. It keeps things flowing.

Let Tech Help You Stay Clear

We often forget that the same technology that clutters us can also organize us if we use it with intention. Try these tools to lighten the mental load:

- **Clean Email:** Automatically filters and tidies your inbox
- **Hazel (Mac):** Automates file organization
- **Freedom / Focus Modes:** Blocks distractions during deep work
- **Notion / Evernote:** Creates an external brain for all your random thoughts and plans
- **Password Managers:** Keep your access secure and simple

Build a tech stack that works like a team; one that lets you do less, not more.

Final Thoughts

Now you have the tools. You've built the muscle. You've done the hard part which was basically getting honest with yourself and reclaiming control. And guess what? That's what digital freedom really looks like. Let's leave the physical cluttered space and turn inwards again; a section I've always cherished – the section that keeps your emotions in check.

Chapter Eight
Clear Heart, Full Self: Detoxing the Feelings That Weigh You Down

Have you ever attempted to go about the house in a heavy winter jacket during mid-summer? That's what emotional clutter feels like. You're carrying things around: old disagreements, unresolved disappointments, guilt, sadness, expectations. And maybe, because they aren't visibly evident, you've convinced yourself that they don't take up space. But they do. They operate undercover.

Emotional clutter is sneaky. It lurks in the borders of our decisions, our reactions, our relationships. It dictates how we are seen, or, sometimes, how we aren't. And, unlike physical clutter, you can't just cram it into a drawer. It follows you into interactions, into your dreams, into the way you interpret silence, tone, and text messages and phew... it's exhausting.

In this chapter, we will now release these emotions so they don't turn into quiet pressure on your chest. We'd be learning the difference between carrying and processing, between holding on and honouring, between suppressing and releasing.

There are healthier ways to hold your story.

Let It Out: A Guided Emotional Release Session

Emotions are not logic puzzles meant to be neatly put away or endlessly analysed. They're meant to move and flow. The ones that stick around the longest are usually the ones we never allowed to leave.

Training yourself to let go of these emotions is giving room for a new decluttered life and you cannot achieve this until you're in control. We're going to walk through three emotional release tools right now. Think of these tools as an internal detoxifier. I've found these tools also convenient for wherever you find yourself so your location doesn't matter. Focus on mastering them instead.

Step 1: Breathe Like You Mean It

I want you to take in huge chunks of air; not just your everyday sigh. We're using the 4-7-8 breathing pattern to help your body feel safe enough to release.

Do this now (or set a 2-minute timer):

1.   Inhale through your nose for 4 seconds
2.   Hold that breath for 7 seconds
3.   Exhale slowly through your mouth for 8 seconds
4.   Repeat 4 times

Pay attention to your shoulders. Are they dropping? Are your thoughts slowing down? You're not "doing it wrong" if your mind wanders. As a matter of fact, you're doing great!

Step 2: Pen-to-Heart Download

Now grab a notebook, a napkin, your notes app, or anything. This is a free-write, which means you don't worry about spelling, grammar, or being "deep." You just write what's there.

Prompt:

"If I could say what I'm really feeling right now without apologising, I'd say..."

Set a timer for 5 minutes. Don't stop writing. Even if it's just, "I don't know what to say." Keep going. Let your subconscious speak. If it turns into a letter to someone (living or gone), let it. If it becomes a list of regrets or confessions or dreams, let it. When you're done, read it back if you want. Or fold it up and tuck it away. Or rip it up. You decide.

Step 3: Move Something Out of You

Emotions live in the body. Sometimes words aren't enough. It's time to let your body finish what your mind has been holding. Choose one of the following - right now:

• **Put on a song that matches your mood.** Let yourself move, sway, dance, stomp.
• **Scream into a pillow.** Or your car. Or the shower.
• **Take a brisk walk.** With no podcast, no phone, no agenda.

- **Cry.** Just let it come. Tears are exits. Let them take something with them.

Set a timer if it helps. Five minutes is enough.

Quick Reflection (1 Minute Max)

Take a breath. Place your hand on your chest if it feels grounding. And ask yourself:

"What do I feel now that I didn't feel 10 minutes ago?"

You don't need a perfect answer. Just notice. That noticing is healing.

You've just decluttered a corner of your emotional attic and you can return to this exercise anytime you feel full inside. The door is always open.

When Stuff Isn't Just Stuff: Letting Go Without Losing Yourself

So there is a part where the physical clutters intersect with our emotional clutters. Remember when we talked about items like photographs or belongings that connected us to our departed ones or to certain memories we could not let go of when treating physical clutters? Well, it was basically because of the emotional attachment we had to these items which are in many ways, a form of emotional clutter themselves.

There's a particular kind of tug in the chest that comes from holding an item you haven't touched in years and still not being able to let it go. It could be anything from a birthday card from someone who's no longer here, a sweater from a chapter of life that feels too far away to revisit, yet too close to release or a box of baby clothes from a child who now towers over you.

However, letting go doesn't mean forgetting. I see it as a means of choosing presence instead of heaviness. So let's carry out the emotional aspects of these physical clutters, bearing in mind that the memory is not stored in the object, but it lives inside you.

So how do you honour the meaning without being buried by the mess?

Tool 1: The Three-Box Method

As you sort through sentimental items, set up three boxes with this in mind, just like the four-box method of the physical declutter:

- **Keep** - Items that still bring genuine warmth or serve an active emotional purpose
- **Digitise and Release** - Take a photo of the item before letting it go. That way, the story stays even if the object doesn't
- **Let Go** - Items you've outgrown emotionally but have held onto out of guilt, obligation, or fear

Take your time. If something feels too loaded, place it aside and don't also trick yourself into believing that every one of such items falls into the keep category. You don't need to rush. Every item released is a little piece of emotional room you gain back.

Tool 2: The One-Year Rule for Sentimental Items

Ask yourself, "Have I interacted with this in the past year?"
If not, go deeper and ask, "If this item were in someone else's home, would I still want it?"

This reframing creates space between your memory and the physical object, helping you decide with more clarity and less guilt. You can thank the item for what it once represented, then take a photo if needed and release it gently.

Tool 3: The "Not Mine" Lens

This insight comes from a community of fellow declutterers I met via a group on Facebook when it was still active in earlier times. When stuck, pretend the item belongs to someone else. Would you still want to keep it? Does it still hold value when stripped of your personal story? This simple trick helps create healthy emotional distance since what stays is the love or lesson, not the thing itself.

The Emotional Four-Box Sort: Making Sense of the Mess in Your Head

Speaking about clutters and boxes, in my journey through emotional healing, I found that emotions could be sorted using the four-box method of physical decluttering. There may just be changes in the label. I see emotional clutter like some sort of physical and mental clutter combined. It leans more towards the mental clutter aspect, though, but just imagine that instead of feeling overwhelmed with being busy, you're always on the verge of tears, telling yourself you're some strong superhero.

It's okay. You're not falling apart. You're just full.

So, what if we used the same idea we apply to sorting out physical clutter to deal with emotional build-up? Instead of "Keep, Donate, Trash," let's bring in a softer, more human-friendly version:

Keep. Let Go. Process Later. Redirect.

Simple enough to remember, deep enough to help you actually feel lighter.
Let's walk through them like we're doing a gentle internal clean-up together.

Keep

These are the thoughts and feelings that are still useful. Maybe it's your love for someone that anchors you or a healthy sense of pride or it's a boundary that still makes sense. You don't need to over-process these - just acknowledge them. They're part of your foundation.
Example: "I'm still proud of how I handled that difficult conversation."
Keep it. It grounds you.

Let Go

Here live the feelings that expired long ago but somehow never got picked up by emotional recycling. Guilt that isn't yours. Shame that came from someone else's judgment. Worry about something that already passed.

Example: "I should've been better back then."

Ask yourself: Does this still serve me, or is it just weighing me down?

If not, let it go. You're allowed.

Process Later

Some feelings are too fresh or too complex to sort right now. That's okay. Don't force them into clarity. Just label them "not now" and come back with more energy and space.

Example: "I don't know why that thing my friend said still bothers me."

You don't need to figure it out in five minutes. You just need to name that it's there and save it for later.

Redirect

These are the spirals, the loops, the thoughts that have become background noise. They might start with something small and end in a rabbit hole of imagined disasters. When you catch one, gently reroute your energy.

Example: "If I don't reply perfectly to this message, they'll think I'm rude."

No need to fight it. Just say, "Not helpful," and give your mind something else to chew on. Music. A walk. A different question.

Emotion-Sorting Activity: Try This in Real Time

Grab a piece of paper. Fold it into four quadrants or label four columns with these headings:
- Keep
- Let Go
- Process Later
- Redirect

Now, write down ten recent thoughts or feelings you've had. Don't censor yourself - messy is okay. Sort each one into its box. Trust your gut. You might be surprised where some of them land.

Art for the Heart: Creative Ways to Let Feelings Move

There were moments when I was opportune to visit a school and have a conversation with some of the children and the class teacher as regards the art subjects. This experience made me understand the level of emotional dump that children put into artistic works. Of course, I had an idea of this before; how children illustrated and communicated their inner recesses and feelings using art but this particular moment was one that made me understand that this craft was not limited to children alone.

Not everything inside you wants to be explained. Some emotions are meant to be expressed through colour, motion, sound, stillness, or imagery that speaks louder than words. Emotional detoxing through creative practices shouldn't necessarily turn you into a painter or a dancer or a wellness guru. And before you begin to feel like you're too grown for this, I'd like you to know that it's still something I do every now and then especially on weekends and whenever I am around kids.

This section is your toolkit, much outlined like mine.

Guided Imagery: Let Your Mind Take You Somewhere Safer

Guided imagery is a tool used in therapy, meditation, and trauma recovery because it works. It engages your imagination and sensory awareness to help your nervous system shift from threat mode into calm. You're giving your brain a new environment; one that signals safety, stillness, and choice.

Let's try a few different visual journeys. You can read them slowly to yourself, record them in your own voice, or ask someone else to read them to you.

Scene 1: The Mountain Cabin

You are standing on the porch of a small wooden cabin high up in the mountains. The air is cool, crisp, and completely still. You can hear the gentle creak of the trees swaying in the wind, the crackle of a fireplace behind you, and the sound of your own breath. You wrap a blanket around your shoulders and breathe deeply. The sky is wide and open. The weight you've been carrying feels like it belongs to someone else. You are safe here.

Scene 2: The Sunlit Field

You walk slowly into a wide, golden field. The grass sways around your knees and the sunlight warms your face. There is no noise, no pressure, no signal. Just you, barefoot, grounded. You drop everything you've been mentally holding onto and watch the breeze carry it away like dandelion seeds. You laugh. Maybe cry a little. But everything feels lighter.

Scene 3: The Ocean Room

You're seated on soft white sand in front of a calm, turquoise ocean. The waves come in and out, slow and steady, like your breathing. You feel each wave pulling away the clutter in your heart: the guilt, the noise, the what-ifs. Every inhale brings in a little peace. Every exhale sends something away.

Choose one. Sit with it for 5–10 minutes. Repeat it whenever emotional noise gets too loud. You don't need the actual location; your mind knows how to build peace inside.

Expressive Art: Draw the Feeling, Not the Thing

Here's the rule: there are no rules.

Forget what you learned in art class. This isn't for public display. It's not for skill. Start with this prompt:

"If my feeling had a shape, a colour, or a pattern, what would it look like?"

Now create it. Use anything: a pencil, highlighter, nail polish, torn magazines. Use coffee to stain the paper. Use lipstick if you have to.

- Rage might look like jagged red lines tearing across the page.
- Sadness might be a puddle of greys and blues.
- Hope might look like gold flecks trying to break through.

Label it if you want. Or don't. Just let it be a map of your inside world. When you're finished, pause. Look at it. Let yourself feel what you created. Then ask:

"Do I feel even one percent lighter?"

If yes, you've done the work.

Movement That Speaks for You

I love dancing, especially when it comes into being used as therapy because it almost always works as not just inner therapy but also physical exercise. If you've ever danced in your room with the door shut and the volume up, you already know the power of this tool. Movement helps finish emotional cycles that thoughts cannot. And you absolutely don't need to be a terrific dancer to carry this out.

Pick your practice:

• **Shake It Out:** Stand in one spot and shake every limb; starting with your arms, then legs, then your whole body. Think of it like loosening stuck energy. Do it for one song.

• **Flow Freely:** Put on a slow instrumental or something ambient. Close your eyes. Let your body decide what to do. Roll your shoulders. Sway. Stretch. Collapse and get back up.

• **Box the Air:** Feeling pent-up anger? Play something hard and fast. Throw punches into the air or into a pillow. Let yourself breathe heavily. You're not fighting. You're releasing.

Music That Mirrors or Moves You

Music bypasses logic and speaks straight to the soul. That's why it's the quickest emotional shortcut available.

Try this:

• **Create an "Emotional Detox" Playlist**

Make four sections or moods:

o   Feel It (songs that let you cry)

o   Shake It Off (songs that get your energy up)

o   Heal It (soft, grounding instrumentals or affirming lyrics)

o   Reclaim It (power songs that remind you who you are)

Let the music take you where you've been afraid to go. And then let it walk you back home.

Vision Boarding: Redirect Emotional Energy with Intention

Once the storm has passed, don't leave the space empty. Fill it with intention. Grab a poster board, a digital canvas, or even just a notebook page. Choose images, words, and colours that represent the emotional state you're moving toward and not away from.

Release Rituals & Farewell Ceremonies

There's another act of emotional self-care that I grew quite fund of, and that is the release ritual. Most times, this is common among those who have lost a loved one as a way of releasing all that grief and heartache. So I gave it a close thought and wondered, "if this ritual worked in letting go of things so dear to us like those we love, how much more other sentimental things to which we've attached meanings that keep us bound?

There's a quiet power in closure. We often think closure happens by accident but we can actually create this closure and comfort ourselves. In this segment, I would relay to you some of the release rituals and farewell ceremonies that have helped me so well in letting go of some of the hurt that bound my emotions and cluttered my feelings.

Why Rituals Matter

Ritual is simply a meaningful action done with attention. It must not be some spiritual act, but attaching spiritual significance most times, gives it more meaning. You don't need candles, incense, or spiritual titles to create one. Once we create a moment to say, "This mattered," we give our hearts permission to loosen their grip.

Here are several release practices you can adapt to your own story:

The Goodbye Letter

I've seen this in quite a number of movies and as much as you want to believe it is just that – movies, it actually does work in ways you can't imagine. Write a letter to the thing (or person or emotion) you're releasing. You can say everything you never got to say - the good, the complicated, the bitter, the soft.

Here's a simple structure to guide you:

• "You came into my life when..."

• "You taught me..."

• "I've carried you because..."

• "But now, I choose to let you go because..."

• "Goodbye, and thank you for..."

You can end the letter however you like. Then, you get to choose what to do with it:

• Tear it up and throw it away.

• Burn it (safely) in a fireproof bowl.

• Bury it under a plant or tree.

• Fold it and store it in a "done" box you'll never reopen.

There's no wrong way to end a letter meant for release.

The Candle Farewell

Light a small candle and sit quietly with it. Think of the emotion or memory you're releasing. You might even say it out loud:

"I'm letting go of the shame I've carried about failing."
"I'm releasing my need for someone's approval."
"I'm saying goodbye to this version of me."

Watch the flame as it burns. When you're ready, blow it out slowly. As the smoke lifts, imagine your emotional weight lifting too. You can repeat this ritual whenever you feel a build-up that words can't untangle.

The Object Goodbye

Some emotional attachments are tethered to physical items. If you're ready to part with it, don't just toss it. Say goodbye with honour.

- Hold the item in your hands.

- Say what it meant to you.

- Acknowledge what you're taking with you and what you're releasing.

Then decide whether you will donate it, bury it, or simply let the ocean carry it... whichever works for you.

The Silent Walk

Pick a short trail, park, or block to walk without accompaniments like music or distractions.

Before you begin, name (quietly or aloud) what you are releasing. With each step, imagine walking farther away from it. You don't need dramatic tears or big moments. Be real within yourself.

At the end of the walk, take one deep inhale. Then exhale slowly and say:

"I'm walking forward. I'm choosing peace."

The Water Release

Water has been symbolic of renewal for centuries. Use it in your ritual.

- Write the name of what you're releasing on a small piece of paper.

- Fold it up and submerge it in a bowl of water.

- As it dissolves or fades, watch your attachment do the same.

- Pour the water out somewhere meaningful. I prefer pouring it into soil.

These rituals won't erase your memories or rewrite your story but they will help you create space for what comes next.

Lifestyle Habits That Quiet the Noise

So someone said the way we eat and our living habits don't count, or perhaps you just feel the topic of health is quite cliché. To be frank, there's no way to discuss declutter without talking about healthy eating and general living habits. Let's get real for a moment. Emotional health doesn't just come from a breakthrough therapy session or a one-off release ritual. Yes, everything we've discussed definitely works but this declutter and detox we are trying to achieve also lives in the boring stuff - like how well you sleep, what you drink when you're stressed, whether you're moving your body, or how often you remember to breathe with both lungs.

It's the daily, quiet habits that build resilience. Let's talk through some of the often-overlooked ways your lifestyle might be either holding you up or holding you back emotionally.

The Sleep Check-In

When was the last time you felt actually rested? Not just "I didn't die in my sleep," but "My brain isn't foggy and I'm not emotionally threadbare by 9 a.m."

Lack of sleep messes with your energy and makes your feelings louder and harder to manage. Sadness feels deeper. Irritation hits harder. Anxiety doesn't shut up.

Try this for a week:

• Set a regular sleep start time (not just a wake-up time).

• Ditch screens 45 minutes before bed.

• Replace the scroll with a small bedtime routine: warm drink, soft lighting, a few pages of a book.

The Hydration Conversation

Weird fact: Emotional overwhelm sometimes feels worse when you're just dehydrated.

I've been there! So start paying attention to what you reach for when you're tired or stressed. Coffee? Wine? Coke? (No judgment.)

Then add a full glass of water first before the other stuff.

Eat to Feel, Not Just Function

You know that one meal that just grounds you? I'm not talking about the fast food band-aid or the bowl of cereal at midnight, but the one that actually makes your body feel calm?
Make more of those.

Setout a routine to include more whole foods, more fibre, and don't forget the joy of eating without rushing or feeling guilty. Include that as well!

Move, Even When You Don't Want To

Emotions get trapped in still bodies. Movement helps metabolise stress hormones. It clears mental fog and brings back the "you" that sometimes disappears under the weight of everything. We've talked about this, but here's just a reminder to make a lifestyle habit out of it: dance in your kitchen, walk the dog, stretch on the floor with a podcast playing.

Go Outside, Like Your Life Depends on It (Because It Kind of Does)

Nature resets the nervous system. Even five minutes outside can lower cortisol levels, boost serotonin, and reduce rumination. So go sit under a tree or water your plants barefoot, watch the clouds move or touch actual dirt. I've once had my teenage phase of staying indoors for so long, drooling and watching time slip by. Believe me, there's no greater way to depression than what the modern generation have now tagged, "introversion."

Self-Care Without the Marketing

Forget bubble baths and luxury candles for a second. Real emotional self-care is:

• Saying no without an essay

• Taking a break before you're broken

• Letting yourself not be productive sometimes

• Asking for help and receiving it like you deserve it (because you do)

Support & Accountability: A Reminder that You Don't Have to Do This Alone

There's a myth we've been fed: that emotional strength means doing it all by yourself. I usually have pity on men the most when it comes to this. "As a man, you have to bottle up your emotions and be strong!" What? Such chaotic belief!

Most emotional clutter doesn't come from weakness but from isolation. You have been holding much, too long, with no safe place to let it land. You must cultivate the mindset of understanding that support doesn't make you needy but human. We all need a shoulder and choosing to share the emotional weight with others - whether through words, presence, or shared experience - is often the missing link in sustainable healing.

Start with Your Circle

Think of one person in your life who holds space well. I'm not talking about the one who tries to fix everything or give unsolicited advice, but the one who listens, nods, and says, "Yeah, that makes sense." If you've found that person, proceed to reaching out. Share a piece of what you're carrying.

You don't need to dump your whole emotional hard drive. As a matter of fact, I'd advise you start small.

"Hey, I've been working on clearing some emotional stuff, and I'm realising how much I hold in. Can I talk something through with you?"

The right people won't run. On the contrary, they'll lean in.

Find or Form a Support Pod

A support pod is a small, trusted group (2–5 people) who check in regularly. You can meet weekly over tea, or create a shared message thread. Use simple prompts:

• What's been emotionally heavy this week?

• What's one thing you're letting go of?

• What do you need support with right now?

When people know they're not alone in the clutter, they become braver about clearing it.

Professional Help Is Not Just for Crises

Therapists, coaches, counsellors - they're not just for when life is falling apart. They're for sorting, naming, processing, and healing in a safe, structured space.

If something keeps resurfacing such as the same fear, anger, or memory, that's a signal and I strongly recommend you see a professional. They can be lifechanging, trust me. You don't have to unpack it alone. A professional gives you tools, perspective, and care without personal entanglement.

If traditional therapy isn't accessible, consider:

• Online therapy platforms (BetterHelp, Talkspace)

• Community centres offering sliding scale support

• University counselling clinics or local NGOs

Online Communities & Anonymous Support

Sometimes it feels easier to share with strangers. That's okay too. Online spaces like Reddit's r/DecidingToBeBetter or mental health Discord servers offer validation without performance.

Use them for:

• Emotional release without judgment

• Getting ideas on what's worked for others

• Feeling seen on your messiest days

Just remember to balance digital vulnerability with real-life connection when possible.

Preventing Emotional Re-Clutter

You've done the work. You've released, reflected, cried a little (or a lot), maybe danced it out in your living room and it goes on but before we go, we need to ensure sustainability. So, like with every other earlier chapter, I'd be providing some tips for maintaining a decluttered emotional.

Daily Emotional Check-Ins

This doesn't need to be a grand ritual. It can be 2–5 minutes each day, just checking your emotional "weather."

As usual, here are daily prompts for you which you can always refer back to:

- What am I feeling right now?
- Where in my body do I feel it?
- Is this feeling new, or familiar?
- Do I need to act on this - or just notice it?

Some people do this in the morning with coffee. Others at night before sleep.

The 3-Minute Emotion Reset

When the day gets noisy or you feel emotionally scrambled, pause. Set a timer for 3 minutes and do this:

1. Sit. Close your eyes if you want.
2. Inhale deeply through your nose for 4 seconds.
3. Hold for 4 seconds.
4. Exhale through your mouth for 6–8 seconds.
5. Repeat.
6. On your last breath, say a word that grounds you: Peace. Here. Enough. Release.

This tiny ritual helps interrupt emotional spirals before they dig in.

Use Affirmations as Emotional Anchors

Affirmations give your brain new scripts to practice. When repeated consistently, they start to replace old mental clutter with intentional thought.

Create a few of your own, or borrow from these:

- "I release what no longer belongs to me."
- "I can feel deeply without drowning."
- "My emotions are signals, not enemies."
- "Today, I choose clarity over chaos."

You can say them aloud, write them on sticky notes, or set them as phone reminders.

Design Your Own Weekly "Emotional Reset"

Once a week, take 15–30 minutes to emotionally check in and reset. This is your time to unclog what's built up quietly over the days.

Here's my template to guide you:

Weekly Emotional Reset (Choose a consistent day/time)

1. How did I feel most of this week?

Tense? Joyful? Overwhelmed? Calm? Numb?

2. What was the emotional high point?

What brought me energy or lightness?

3. What was the emotional low point?

What drained me, and why?

4. What emotional clutter am I holding that I can release now?

A grudge? A mistake? A "should" that no longer fits?

5. One act of self-kindness I'll offer myself this week:

Something nourishing, restorative, or joyful.

We've been through quite the emotional journey, but we're not done with what lies inwards. The next chapter will take us even deeper; into what lies not just inward, but beyond!

Chapter Nine
A Lighter Spirit: Making Room for Meaning in a Noisy World

Among the different types of detox exercises, the spiritual detox is the most ignored; at least I believe this to be so. Many people ignore the fact that beyond what we see in the physical world, there is a spiritual layer to everything at play; one that we are meant to access to control the eventualities of the real world. Now, the funny thing is that you don't have to believe in anything lofty or cosmic to feel like something's missing. Sometimes, the heaviness isn't emotional or mental, but something deeper. You look around at your life and wonder why even the good things feel a bit muted. It may be time to dive deeper into the spiritual aspect.

This chapter is not one I have drafted for religion fanatics to explore spirituality from the light of their individual beliefs. As a matter of fact, we'd be clearing the inner noise, the inherited beliefs, the routines that don't match who you are anymore, and finding your way back to something that feels simple and sacred. Of course, you can hold on to your religious beliefs; nothing we'd be discussing here tampers with them in any way. This is just my neutral way of spiritual detox that can apply to anyone, irrespective of what you believe in.

The Practice of Mindfulness

The mind is not the brain; it goes much deeper than that. For me, it's a spiritual projection of our mentality and mindfulness is the key to attaining control of the mind. Different people have different ideas around being mindful but for me, it is simply learning to notice what's happening right here, right now, without automatically reacting and in spiritual detoxing, that act of noticing has power. It becomes a way to let go of outdated stories, emotional habits, and inner noise that clutters your deeper sense of meaning.

What Mindfulness Actually Means

Mindfulness is the ability to focus your attention gently on your breathing, your body, and the moment you are in, and then step back from judgment or mental storylines about what you "should" be feeling or doing. Secular programs like MBSR (Mindfulness-Based Stress Reduction) define it as nonjudgmental awareness of thoughts, emotions, and bodily sensations, practiced moment by moment. Instead of trying to empty your mind, you learn to observe what moves through it and let it pass without carrying it with you.

Research shows that regular mindfulness practice strengthens neural pathways associated with focus, emotional resilience, and stress regulation. It reduces anxiety, improves mood, and helps break patterns of rumination or reactivity. In clinical settings, mindfulness is now widely accepted as a valuable, evidence-based tool for mental and spiritual wellness.

How Mindfulness Fuels Inner Detox

Over time, unexamined beliefs, recurring anxieties, inherited expectations, or spiritual shame settle into our emotional landscape. Mindfulness functions like a gentle filter that clears that sediment.

When you notice your breath, your body, even a recurring thought about "not being enough," you begin to reclaim it from unconscious control. You stop reacting and start choosing. This shift is profoundly spiritual without needing faith and just needing attention and an open mind.

Mindfulness Practice Basics

Here are four key principles to guide a spiritual mindfulness practice:

1. Intention: Begin by anchoring your attention with purpose. That could be a phrase like "I want presence" or "I want clarity," or simply a resolve to observe without judgement.

2. Attention: Notice your breath, body sensations, or thoughts. If

your mind wanders, gently bring it back without criticism.

3. Non-judging: Emotions or thoughts labelled "good" or "bad" tend to create more inner clutter. Mindfulness invites you to just see them without adding commentary.

4. Ethical awareness: Mindfulness also invites a broader awareness of your interactions like what you consume, how you speak, and how you act. It connects presence with purpose.

A Simple Mindfulness Practice You Can Try Now

•   Sit in a chair or lie down, make sure you're comfortable, and close your eyes if you want.

•   Take slow breaths for one minute, counting four seconds in, holding two, and exhaling for six.

•   After a minute, notice where attention is: your chest rising, your mind drifting, a sound outside.

•   Whatever you notice, say gently in your mind: "Noticing..." or "Here it is..." and then ease your attention back to the breath.

Start with three to five minutes, once or twice a day. Even brief daily practice reshapes how your mind responds under stress and invites emotional clarity over time. It totally worked for me.

Interactive Activity: A Week of Mindful Moments

Choose one of these mindfulness practices and do it each day for seven days. Write down how you feel before and after.

• Body scan: Lie or sit quietly and move your attention slowly from your toes to your head, noticing any tension or sensation in each part.

• Mindful walking: Take five slow steps, paying full attention to what your feet feel, the ground beneath you, any sounds or smells around.

• Breath check-ins: At midday, stop for a minute and simply watch your breathing, not changing it and just noticing its rhythm.

• Mindful task: Do one routine activity like washing dishes, eating, or brushing teeth with full presence. Notice the sensations.

After each session take two minutes to journal: "What showed up that surprised me? What did I learn?"

Soul-Cleaning Practices for Everyday Life

When I come across certain situations and make certain decisions, one vital question I always asked myself was, "does this make sense for who I am becoming?" Spiritual clutter is something you have to consciously keep track of because a large part of it is neither dramatic nor visible. It instead builds slowly from your outdated beliefs, autopilot routines, unresolved inner stories, and life choices that no longer reflect your current values. So, for me, soul-cleaning is a form of spiritual cleansing using guided steps that are very practicable, much like those we have carried out in our emotional detox exercises but now with a different target in mind.

Let's look at some practical and reflective ways to do this.

Prompt-Based Journaling for Spiritual Alignment

The idea here is to put your internal world in front of you, using questions that pull your awareness out of routine and back into purpose. Here are a few prompts that are simple but surprisingly revealing when answered regularly:

• "Does this habit/thought/belief align with the kind of life I want to live?"
• "Where in my day do I feel most disconnected from myself?"
• "What area of my life feels heavy and what do I believe is causing that?"
• "What would I release right now if I believed I was allowed to change?"
• "Which part of my identity feels inherited, not chosen?"

You can journal with any of these questions in the morning to set your direction, or at night to take inventory. Like I always say, feel free to have your answers be messy, honest, and even contradictory if needed.

Guided Visualization: Releasing Outdated Inner Stories

Just as mental narratives can lead to mental and emotional clutters, it can also cause spiritual clutters if not properly managed. Mental narratives of who we are, where we emerge from and what will become of us have been formed early or passed on by others. These narratives have deeper meanings in our life than you imagine. In fact, you must be very careful of the kind of stories or beliefs you put your mind to. Some stories help us grow; others quietly limit us. This practice helps bring those stories into view so you can decide whether to keep, rewrite, or release them.

Try this visual exercise:
• Sit quietly. Close your eyes. Take three slow, deep breaths.
• Imagine a hallway with four doors. Each door holds a story you've been told about yourself - maybe something like "I have to always be the strong one," or "Success only counts if others approve," or "I can't be both kind and powerful."
• One by one, open each door and step inside. Notice what the story feels like. Is it heavy? Is it warm? Does it still feel true?
• Now walk out of the story. Gently close the door. You're not erasing it. You're acknowledging that it doesn't define you anymore.
• At the end of the hallway is a new door. When you open it, there's no script; just light. Step into that space and stand there for a moment. Ask yourself, "What am I free to believe now?"
You can write about this experience afterward or revisit it anytime you feel stuck in an old version of yourself.

Activity: The Soul-Clean Sweep

This practice is a reset button for a specific area of your life; a way to turn off autopilot, zoom out, and see where you may have spiritually or emotionally checked out. The idea is to pick one area and examine it with fresh eyes.

Here's how to do it:

Step 1: Choose a Focus Area

Pick just one:

- Your morning routine
- Your job or work mindset
- Your digital habits
- A close relationship
- Your spiritual practices

Step 2: Ask the Core Questions

Use these reflection questions to sweep out what's stagnant:

- "How do I currently feel about this part of my life?"
- "What parts of this are life-giving?"
- "What feels obligatory, hollow, or disconnected?"
- "Am I doing this out of habit, fear, guilt, or alignment?"

Step 3: Identify One Shift

Now, choose one small but intentional adjustment:

- A new boundary (e.g., "No checking emails before 9am.")
- A reframe (e.g., "This isn't failure - this is redirection.")
- A dropped task (e.g., "I no longer need to say yes to everything.")
- A new intention (e.g., "I will start each morning with stillness, not scrolling.")

Write your shift on a note and keep it visible for the next 7 days.

Optional Challenge: Commit to doing a Soul-Clean Sweep each week for a month; one area per week. At the end of the month, journal about how you feel. What stayed the same? What subtly shifted?

Let's get into it.

Curating What Feeds the Soul

As much as you give the physical body the nourishment it needs by eating, so does the spiritual form rely on certain contents to stay healthy. Most people don't realise just how much of their emotional and spiritual clutter comes from what they consume. I'm not really talking about doomscrolling or news overload this time; though those absolutely count. I'm talking about everything you take in without thinking like the podcast you half-listen to on auto-pilot, the friend's daily complaints that leave you feeling drained, the music you play without noticing how it affects your mood, the routines you repeat even though they no longer bring joy.

Every input either feeds you or empties you.

That's why spiritual must entail choosing deliberately what you let in; let the keyword for you be "deliberately." What lifts you? What aligns with your deeper values? What energises the quiet parts of you that usually go ignored? I remember how often I listened to these sad songs in those carefree youthful days and just how much impact it had on me.

Let's get really practical about this.

The Soul Audit: Inspired vs. Drained

Grab a notebook or open a digital note and divide the page in two. Label one side **Feeds Me**, and the other **Drains Me**. Then take a few minutes to honestly list things under each heading:

- What kinds of content do you scroll through?
- What conversations leave you recharged vs. depleted?
- What routines bring you lightness, and which ones feel like obligation?
- What kind of media (music, shows, social feeds, books) are you letting shape your emotional atmosphere?

You might find surprises. Maybe that motivational podcast you used to love now feels pushy and performance-driven. Maybe a YouTube channel about slow living sparks more peace in five minutes than a whole day of hustle content. Maybe your morning silence with tea feeds you more than any advice ever could. Get all these straight and do yourself the favour of being honest with it all.

The One Habit Challenge

Once you're clear on what feeds you, the next step is choosing one daily habit that actively nourishes your inner world. Just one. You may be able to take on more than one at a time, but I prefer beginning with smaller measures. Here are a few soul-feeding ideas to consider:

• A 10-minute walk
• Playing an old song you loved as a teenager
• Lighting a candle while journaling to create a moment of stillness
• Sketching or doodling without a goal
• Sitting outside and watching the sky for a couple quiet minutes
• Preparing one meal mindfully

Pick one and commit to doing it every day for the next 7 days. Set a daily reminder if you need to. Not to force it, but to make space for it.

Activity: Your Soul Feeding Plan

Use this framework to guide your own intentional curation of daily inputs:

Category	What Drains Me	What Feeds Me	One Change I'll Make
Content	Mindless scrolling on Twitter	Listening to instrumental music	Replace scrolling with music at lunch
People	Group chats that feel negative	Weekly call with my sister	Leave one draining group chat
Routine	Starting my day with email	Morning stretch + tea	10-minute screen-free morning
Environment	Cluttered workspace	A clear table with a plant	Tidy desk at end of day

You can update this plan weekly, monthly, or seasonally. Treat it like a living document that reflects your evolving needs.

Sacred Togetherness

Christians go to churches, Muslims go to the mosques and it goes on and on; each sect with a meeting place. Not everyone finds spiritual meaning in the same places. For some, and I'm talking people like me, it's found in stillness. For others, it's found in movement, music, or simply in the company of someone who gets it even when no words are spoken. These are some of the many ways we establish communion. Here's something that holds true across nearly every form of human spirituality: we are wired for connection.

When it comes to spiritual decluttering, I find this communion a vital part of the journey, as it was for me. This doesn't require a shared belief system or rituals or anything outwardly. It can begin in a living room, over a kitchen table, or sitting on a park bench beside someone who's willing to go a little deeper than "how's your week been?" What makes a moment spiritually nourishing isn't formality but intentionality.

Spiritual community, when stripped of hierarchy and pressure, becomes an offering: "I'll hold space for you if you'll hold space for me."

What Non-Religious Spiritual Connection Looks Like

You don't need to label anything sacred for it to carry weight. Here are a few forms of shared experience that foster spiritual clarity and warmth without a need for shared doctrine:

• Paired Reflection: You can sit with someone and take turns answering a few simple, open-ended questions. What's something you're working through quietly? What brought you joy this week that no one else noticed? What belief about yourself is changing?

• Group Art Sessions: Another moment to discuss art as a whole. Get a few friends together with paints, markers, collage materials and a theme. "What does renewal feel like?" "What am I letting go of?" Create without critique. Let the process do the talking.

• Symbolic Acts of Service: Pick something simple but meaningful to do together like writing notes of encouragement for strangers, planting something, or creating a shared journal you pass between one another.

• Silent Companionship: Yes, it's a thing. So you can sit side by side with a friend and read, breathe, draw, or write without talking. Agree on a time boundary. Just the presence of another person in stillness with you can feel incredibly expansive.

• Shared Ritual Creation: Instead of following one, make your own. It could be a monthly reflection dinner where everyone brings one "light" and one "weight" or a candle-lighting ritual on the last Sunday of the month, or perhaps, a "release box" where friends anonymously drop what they're letting go of.

Host a Shared "Soul Clean-Out" Session

I want you to imagine something a little different from your usual hangout. How about you have just you and one or two people you trust, coming together not to fix anything, but to make space. Trust me, in this form of company, your soul gets a bit of room to breathe.

Start by inviting someone
Though you want to do this to heal, you don't necessarily need the people around to be those types of people that turn everything into a therapy session either. For me, I just find someone who makes me feels safe. Invite someone you can laugh with, or sit beside without needing to fill the silence. I've found that one or two people is the sweet spot; enough to not feel alone, small enough to keep it intimate.

Now set the space
You don't have to go full retreat-mode. It could be your living room, the porch, or a quiet corner of a park. I like to change one small thing to make it feel intentional, like maybe we sit on cushions instead of the couch, or I light a candle or put on music that doesn't ask for attention. Water or tea in mugs always helps because it

160

gives your hands something to hold. All these together also signals to your brain that this moment is a little different.

Here's how we begin

I usually say something simple like, "I just want us to have a space where we can let go of anything we've been dragging around." Then I offer some gentle prompts. Sometimes just one question opens up something real.

Try these:

• What's something I've been holding that I no longer need?
• What part of my story feels like it's ready for a rewrite?
• Where do I feel spiritually tired and what would refresh me?
• What's one thing I want more of in my life, and what's been blocking it?

I prefer you just discuss and talk about your answers and zero your mind on expectations. Sometimes the best moments happen when someone says, "I'm not sure yet," and we sit with that.

End gently. Don't rush off

I like closing with a small act as well. Maybe we write down one thing we're ready to release and tear the paper together. Or we speak a word - just one - that we want to carry into the next week. Something like "ease" or "trust" or "pause." You could even choose a shared word as a group and let that be your quiet anchor.

The whole thing doesn't need to be longer than an hour. Everything together is just to remind yourself that you're not carrying everything alone that letting something go can happen in the most ordinary of spaces, with people who simply show up.

Maintaining Spiritual Space

Decluttering, in any form, is never just a one-time event as we've gotten to understand even from earlier chapters. It is a relationship between you and your inner life that you have to keep in constant maintenance. Don't be fooled by the mere practicality of it and just see it as nothing. The peace of your entire life hangs in the balance and just like any relationship worth keeping, it needs a rhythm that can flow with your life and adjusts with your seasons.

So let's explore ways we can constantly avoid spiritual clutter by maintaining the space after decluttering.

Monthly Mini-Retreats: Reset Before the Rush

Once a month (preferably the first Sunday or the last Friday for me), set aside a half-day, or even just two quiet hours, where you unplug from output and tune into yourself.

Use the time to reflect, journal, or revisit your emotional or spiritual journey so far. Maybe you reread an entry in your journal, light a candle, or listen to music that brings you back to center. I keep mentioning the basic habits because as I have experienced, it's so easy to do these every day.

Daily Micro-Rituals: Moments, Not Movements

We all have a morning routine, even if it's messy. At some point in my life, my morning ritual was just doodling. Yes, it gets that awkward. Your micro-ritual might look like:

- Taking three breaths with your hand over your heart before you speak to anyone
- Whispering a word of the day to yourself like "patience," "flow," "listen"
- Lighting a match or incense stick as a signal that you're starting the day with awareness
- Washing your hands slowly while thinking about what you're releasing
- Or simply doing what everyone does – cleaning your teeth!

Activity: Draft Your Spiritual Declutter Calendar

We can do this easily without making a big show of it so save it; you won't be needing a spreadsheet. Let's get on that piece of paper and write down some meaning!

1. **Pick your day**

Choose one day a month that feels least chaotic. Write it down as your Spiritual Check-in Day. Set a gentle reminder. This is your mini-retreat anchor.

2. Name your weekly pulse

Choose one small thing you'll do every week to reset. It could be a 10-minute walk in silence on Sundays, journaling on Friday nights, or even pulling a single word card on a Monday morning.

3. Design your micro-daily

Choose one tiny act to repeat daily, like, perhaps, placing your hand on your chest when you wake up or looking at the sky for one minute before you sleep.

4. Leave space to evolve

Life shifts so you can always let your calendar breathe. Add, remove, and change your rituals as needed.

Part III
The Full Life

**"...The energy it takes to hang onto the past
is holding you back from a new life."**
- Mary Manin Morrissey

Chapter Ten
Focus Is the New Freedom

You've come a long way, revolving around all five sectors of a decluttering journey. If you had successfully carried out or you're still carrying out the tasks in each of the earlier chapters, then you should give yourself a pat on the back. It's nothing easy. It took several years for me to fully understand what it meant and took to do a thorough run through of my entire life. I can imagine it was so for me because I definitely didn't have a book like this that gathered all the information I needed into one place to guide me.

However, with such book now present and all my years of knowledge now brought together in one place as this, I do hope it has gone a long way for you. Now, for a final closing and to put a seal on everything we've explored together, I shall now be giving you the very last element you need to make it all complete, and that is focus!

Now, take a deep breath. We've done so much; here, we won't be using that much intensity. We're done through the difficult part. Let's now go through that seamless part that crowns it all like the cherry on the cake.

The Idea of True Focus

What does it actually mean to be focused? It depends on how you want to look at it. For this case scenario, though, I'm exploring the idea of having a life focus.

Focus in life means giving your full attention to what truly matters and tuning out everything else.

In a practical sense, it's deciding on a goal and pouring your energy into it without letting distractions pull you away. In fact, focus is like the engine that turns your plans into reality meaning it aligns your attention with your intention and transforms raw effort into real results. When you stay focused on one task or goal at a time, you're able to make genuine progress instead of scattering your efforts in all directions. In today's world of constant pings and notifications, this kind of dedicated attention has become both challenging and extremely valuable.

Most of us were raised on the idea that success is about expanding; that is doing more, achieving more, being more. However, somewhere along the way, all that "more" started costing us something we didn't realise was negotiable: our peace of mind. In our present time, we confuse busyness for purpose. We chase opportunity like it's going out of stock. We say yes just in case and in doing so, we throw things like our health, presence, joy, depth out the window.

Focus shouldn't be, for you, the art of doing less because you've failed to keep up. It's about doing less *on purpose*. It is like, out of the complex mix, you're deciding to pick what matters most and let it be enough.

You don't need to do everything; you just need to do the right things, and by that, I mean the ones that are right *for you*. And that's what we're about to work through together.

Curating True Focus in Life

One of the first steps to building better focus is being clear about your goals and priorities. If you don't know exactly what you want, it's easy to drift aimlessly without getting anything significant done. Think of **clarity** as having a roadmap – when your objectives are well-defined, you can make informed decisions about how to spend your time and energy. For example, if your goal is to write a book, breaking it down into specific milestones (like writing one chapter per week) gives you a clear target to focus on. Without that clarity, you might find yourself procrastinating or getting sidetracked, but with it, you can channel your actions toward something meaningful.

Along with clear goals comes **prioritization**: not everything on your plate is equally important, so focusing means identifying the tasks that matter most and putting them first. You might have a long to-do list, but effective focus is about zooming in on the one or two things that will advance your goals the most and tackling those first. By consciously saying "yes" to what's important (and "no" to what's not), you make sure your limited time and energy go into the things that truly count.

Of course, even with clear goals, distractions are everywhere. We've all had moments where we sit down to work on something important and then a phone notification or a random thought derails us for half an hour. Part of developing focus is **minimizing** these distractions and training yourself to be mentally present. That might mean silencing your phone, closing unnecessary browser tabs, or finding a quiet space to work. It could also involve managing internal distractions, like those anxious thoughts about the future or dwelling on past mistakes.

Bear in mind that focus is easiest when you're living in the **present moment**, fully engaged in what you're doing right now because in all honesty, that's what matters. A useful insight here is that focus isn't just about doing more; it's often about doing less – specifically, doing less of the unimportant stuff.

Productivity expert James Clear put it nicely: *"Focus is the art of knowing what to **ignore**."* In practice, that means intentionally ignoring the notifications, temptations, and side-tasks that aren't serving your goal. For example, if you're working on an important report, you might decide to ignore email for an hour and avoid checking social media. By deliberately choosing what not to pay attention to, you free up your mind to concentrate on the task at hand. This selective attention can unlock greater clarity and efficiency in your work. It's worth noting that science backs this up – when you allow yourself to be interrupted, it can take a long time to regain your concentration. One study found that after a typical distraction (say, checking a message), it takes over 23 minutes to get back into a deep focus on the original task. That's a huge loss of time and momentum. So, minimizing interruptions isn't just a personal preference, it's really crucial if you want to maintain high productivity and flow.

Staying focused consistently requires **discipline and persistence**. It's not a one-time choice you make, but a habit you have to cultivate day after day. Even people with clear goals and the best intentions will face moments when focusing is hard – maybe the work gets challenging or boredom sets in, or there's a setback that makes you want to give up. This is where persistence comes in. Focus means coming back to your priority again and again, even after your mind wanders or things go wrong.

In a way, focus is a series of continuous decisions: every time you notice your attention drifting, you gently steer it back to what matters. As one leadership coach put it, *"Focus isn't just about ignoring distractions. It's about deciding, again and again, what matters most, and giving it your full attention."* In practical terms, building this kind of discipline might involve creating routines and environments that support your concentration. For instance, you could set aside specific blocks of time in your day dedicated to your most important work (sometimes called "deep work" or focus time) and treat those like appointments that nothing should interrupt. Some people develop rituals, like turning off all notifications when it's focus time, or using techniques like the Pomodoro method (working in concentrated 25-minute bursts). These little strategies and habits reinforce your commitment to focus. Over time, they train your brain to get into a concentrated state more easily and stay there longer. It's similar to working out a muscle; the more consistently you practice focusing, the stronger your attention span gets.

Why You Need Focus In Your Life

Developing better focus brings a ton of benefits that can genuinely improve your work and life. First off, there's the obvious boost in **productivity**. When you concentrate on one thing at a time, you tend to get more done in less time. You're not wasting minutes (or hours) switching back and forth between tasks, so all that energy is directed like a laser beam. It's common to find that a task which might take all day when you're distracted can be finished in an hour or two of solid focus.

The work you do is often **higher quality** as well, because by giving it your full attention, you catch the details and make fewer mistakes. Think about a time when you were fully "in the zone" working on something – you probably did it better than when you were half-distracted, right? Focused individuals have been found to be not only more productive but even more innovative in their thinking because they're deeply engaged with the problem or project at hand. When you're truly dialled in, you can find creative solutions more easily, since your mind has the space to explore one topic deeply instead of skimming many things superficially.

Plus, naturally, staying focused helps you reach your goals **faster**. Every bit of effort you invest goes toward actual progress on your goal, so you tend to hit milestones and complete projects more consistently. It's a simple equation:

consistent focus = consistent progress

Many big achievements in careers or personal endeavours boil down to regular focused work. Whether it's advancing in a profession, writing a novel, getting in shape, or any other goal, those who stick with a focused routine often see results while others who scatter their efforts do not.

Another huge benefit of focus is its impact on your **mental well-being and personal growth**. Ironically, focusing on fewer things can make life feel less stressful. When you have a clear plan and you're concentrating on one task at a time, you avoid that overwhelming feeling of having too many tabs open in your brain. Instead of stressfully juggling multiple responsibilities at once, you give yourself permission to deal with them one by one. This approach can reduce anxiety and the sense of being overloaded because you know you're handling the important stuff in an orderly way.

Focus can also bring a sense of **calm and control**; you're actively managing your attention rather than feeling pulled in every direction. Plus, with focus, you often get to finish things - and checking off meaningful tasks is rewarding and confidence-building, which further eases stress.

Moreover, when you focus deeply, you tend to learn and **absorb information much better**. Imagine trying to study a new language while also watching TV versus studying in a quiet room with full attention – the latter is clearly more effective. Concentration allows you to dive deeper into subjects, leading to insights and understanding that you'd likely miss if your mind was elsewhere. In fact, being deeply focused can sometimes lead to a mental state known as "flow," where you become so immersed in an activity that you lose track of time and find the work intrinsically rewarding. In a flow state, people often perform at their peak and learn new skills or information at a much faster rate because they're fully engaged. Reaching this state isn't an everyday thing, but it shows how powerful sustained focus can be for personal development and creativity.

Finally, there's the benefit of a **greater sense of purpose and direction** in life. We'd be talking more about this shortly though. When you consistently focus on your true priorities – the goals and values that matter most to you – your daily actions start aligning with your long-term aspirations. Instead of feeling like you're just drifting or busy with *"stuff"* that doesn't matter, you feel more purpose-driven. Each day has direction because you know why *you're doing* what you're doing. Over time, this alignment of focus and purpose can make your life feel more meaningful. You're not just reacting to whatever comes at you; you're proactively building the life or career you want, one focused step at a time.

Purpose in Life: A Practical Overview

Have you ever wondered why you jump out of bed in the morning and what truly keeps you going? That "why" – the reason behind all those early mornings and hard work – is essentially your purpose in life. In simple terms, your purpose is the reason for your existence or the big **"why"** that drives your decisions and actions. It gives you a sense of direction and meaning, making even the tough days feel worthwhile. When you have a clear purpose, you feel that your life has significance and that you're working toward something that matters.

This purpose can come from many places. For some people, it's closely tied to their **vocation** or career – especially if they love what they do or feel their work contributes to the greater good. For others, it might stem from a personal **passion** or a deep desire to contribute to something larger than themselves, like a community, a family, or a cause.

Personal Meaning and Goals

Finding a life purpose often starts with finding **personal meaning** in your experiences and setting meaningful goals. It's about looking at what truly matters to you and creating something valuable out of it. In fact, psychologists often define purpose as **"an abiding intention to achieve a long-term goal that is both personally meaningful and makes a positive mark on the world"**. In other words, your purpose usually isn't a short-term aim – it's more like a long-term guiding star that you're continually working toward because it deeply matters to you. This sense of purpose can become a guiding light for how you live your life. When you know what your big "why" is, it naturally influences your choices and behavior. You'll find that you tend to set goals that align with that purpose and steer away from things that don't.

For example, if your life purpose centers around **creativity**, you might choose a career in the arts or set aside regular time for creative hobbies. In day-to-day life, you'll probably make decisions that nurture your creative spirit – like taking an art class or spending time in inspiring environments – because those choices support your purpose. In this way, having a clear purpose guides you, helping you stay focused on what's important and making it easier to decide what to do (and what not to do) as you move forward.

Contributing to Something Larger

A powerful aspect of life purpose is that it often involves **contributing to something larger than yourself**. Many people find their purpose is linked to how they can help others or make a positive difference in the world around them. There's a special fulfilment that comes from knowing you're impacting someone else's life in a good way. Maybe your purpose is caring for your family, supporting your friends, or improving your community – whatever it is, it likely connects you to others. Often, this aspect of purpose can tie into your career or daily activities. If you can align your work with your values and desire to help, it can give you a strong sense of purpose and satisfaction.

Examples of Purpose in Action:

- **Volunteering:** You might volunteer at a local shelter or community center, using your time and skills to improve others' lives.
- **Mentoring:** Perhaps you find meaning in guiding or teaching others – for instance, mentoring a younger person in your field or helping kids in your neighbourhood learn and grow.
- **Creative Endeavours:** If you're an artist, writer, or innovator, you could pursue creative projects that inspire people or bring joy and insight to others.
- **Advocacy and Causes:** You might dedicate yourself to a cause, like protecting the environment or standing up for social justice, because you're driven to make the world better.

These are just a few ways purpose can manifest. The common thread is that living with purpose often involves reaching beyond your own needs and positively affecting someone or something else. When you see the impact of your actions on others, it often reinforces that sense of purpose even more.

A Journey, Not a Destination

It's important to remember that discovering and living your purpose is a **journey, not a one-time destination**. In fact, your sense of purpose can evolve and change throughout your life as you grow, learn, and go through new experiences. What motivates you or feels deeply meaningful in your twenties might shift by the time you reach middle age or older – and that's completely normal.

For example, you might start out feeling that your purpose is tied to **building a career**, and later on, you realize it has more to do with **family** or **community** (or vice versa). Purpose isn't static; it can adapt as you do. The key is to stay open and willing to explore what matters to you at each stage of life. Think of finding purpose as a continuous process of self-discovery: you keep learning about yourself and what gives you that spark of meaning, and you adjust your path accordingly. Since life is always changing, we sometimes have to **revisit and renew** our sense of purpose when we hit major transitions (like graduation, career changes, retirement, etc.) so that our life direction stays aligned with our current values and passions.

Another thing to note is how having a strong sense of purpose helps you handle life's ups and downs. Life isn't always easy – we all face challenges, setbacks, and moments of doubt. During those tough times, purpose acts like a north star or a steady compass. When you know why you're doing what you're doing, it gives you resilience. Research has found that people who feel a clear sense of purpose tend to cope better with stress and even enjoy better health and well-being overall. It makes sense: if you believe your life has meaning and you're working toward something important, you can endure a lot more. Instead of getting completely discouraged by obstacles, you might say to yourself, "This is hard right now, but it's worth it because I'm working toward **X**." In this way, purpose provides strength and motivation to push through difficulties – it helps you bounce back and keep going when things get tough.

Finding Your Purpose

So, how do you go about finding your own purpose in life? There's no one-size-fits-all answer, because everyone's journey is personal. However, there are some practical steps and reflections that can help you uncover what truly drives you. Here are a few tips to get you started:

• **Reflect on your strengths and values:** Take some time to think about what you're good at and what truly matters to you. What activities make you feel alive or satisfied? What values (like creativity, helping others, independence, etc.) do you hold dear? Understanding your passions, skills, and core values is a big first step in pinpointing a meaningful direction.

• **Seek inspiration from others:** Look at the people you admire or who inspire you. What about their lives or work resonates with you? Sometimes hearing stories of how others found their purpose – whether it's a mentor, a public figure, or a friend – can spark ideas for your own path. You might even talk to mentors or people you trust about how they discovered what mattered to them.

• **Engage with your interests:** Try doing more of the things that naturally draw your interest or curiosity. If you've always felt curious about a subject or activity, dive in deeper. For example, if you care about helping people, maybe volunteer for a project in your community. If you love music or art, take a class or join a group. Experiencing different activities can help you discover what feels most meaningful to you in practice.

• **Be patient and persistent:** Finding your purpose is a journey that can take time – and that's okay. It's normal to feel a bit unsure or to try a few different paths before something clicks. Be patient with yourself and keep exploring. Pay attention to what experiences give you a sense of fulfilment or pride. Over time, patterns will emerge. And remember, your purpose can evolve; what's important is that at any given moment, you keep moving toward the things that give you a sense of meaning and joy, even if it's in small steps.

Finally, keep in mind that your purpose doesn't have to be something grandiose or globally recognized. It just has to be meaningful to you. It could be raising a loving family, spreading kindness in your daily interactions, creating art that moves people, or running a business that solves a problem. Big or small, if it gives you a reason to get up in the morning and makes you feel that your life has meaning, it counts. Embrace the process of finding and living your purpose – it's a personal adventure that can bring a deeper sense of fulfilment to your life. And as you grow and change, don't be afraid to redefine your purpose. Staying true to what matters most to you will help guide you, no matter what life throws your way.

A Brief Farewell

We've come a long way, and at this point, I'm just going to leave you to it, because to be honest, the moment you finish this book is when the job actually begins. I have worked and accumulated the knowledge I have culminated into this book over several years. You don't need to scamper around anymore, trying to discover what works.

You just need to declutter!

As overwhelming as it may appear to be, decluttering is just basic tidying up (litotes intended). But really, you're basically noticing what you're carrying, deciding what's worth keeping, and making space for what actually matters. The emails, the childhood mementos, the cluttered to-do lists, the expectations, the quiet heaviness you couldn't always name - it's all connected. And in facing it piece by piece, you've made something bigger than space. You've made clarity. You've made a decision that will live with you for the rest of your life!

Now, look at this secret I'll leave you with.

There will still be clutter. That's life.

I once visited my sister and after a year, I returned to her home to find that many of the items I used like the cloth hangers and the likes, we're stuffed somewhere, feeding on dust. I simply saw one thing – growth. There was now an even better alternative to those hangers. Your clutter can be a sign of growth. Still, it could be a weapon of your downfall if you don't properly plan your life.

But now, you've got the tools to pause, reassess, and reset. You've built a new kind of rhythm - one that gives you room to breathe, to feel, to create, to rest, and to grow.

And the best part? You did it by starting exactly where you were.

So, whatever comes next, remember: the space is yours. You've earned it.

References

Alyssa Longobucco (2025, June 27). 5 Items You Absolutely MUST Toss in Your Bathroom, According to Pro Organizers. House Beautiful. https://www.housebeautiful.com/lifestyle/organizing-tips/a65193562/things-in-bathroom-to-throw-out-professional-organizers/

Asurion. (2019). Americans check their phones 96 times a day. https://www.asurion.com/connect/tech-tips/phone-usage/

Baratan, A. (2025, July 4). How to Declutter a Small Kitchen - 10 Tips for Clearing Out. Livingetc. https://www.livingetc.com/advice/how-to-declutter-a-small-kitchen

Baumeister, R. F. (1991). Meanings of life. Guilford Press.

Baumeister, R. F., & Tierney, J. (2011). Willpower: Rediscovering the Greatest Human Strength. Penguin Press.

Carr, N. (2010). The shallows: What the internet is doing to our brains. W.W. Norton & Company.

Carver, C. (2015). How to Let Go of Sentimental Items. Be More with Less. https://bemorewithless.com/victorylap/

Chen, V. (2024, April 24). Inbox Zero: A Guide to Clearing Your Email Clutter. UseMotion Blog. https://www.usemotion.com/blog/inbox-zero

Clear, J. (2018). Atomic Habits. Avery.

Clear, J. (2018). Atomic Habits (Chapter 12 excerpt: "How to Make Your Future Habits Easy"). https://jamesclear.com/reset-the-room

Csikszentmihalyi, M. (1990). Flow: The Psychology of Optima Experience. Harper & Row.

Damásio, H., & Damásio, A. R. (2016). Exploring the construction of the conscious self through purpose. Greater Good Science Center. https://greatergood.berkeley.edu

Daminger, A. (2019). The cognitive dimension of household labor. American Sociological Review, 84(4), 609–633. https://doi.org/10.1177/0003122419859007

Flinders University Student Health & Wellbeing. (n.d.). What is life purpose? https://blogs.flinders.edu.au/student-health-and-well-being/2020/09/01/what-is-life-purpose

Frankl, V. E. (1984). Man's search for meaning (Rev. ed.). Washington Square Press.

Fuller, K. (2023, August 21). How clutter and mental health are connected. Verywell Mind. https://www.verywellmind.com/decluttering-our-house-to-cleanse-our-minds-5101511

Goleman, D. (2013). Focus: The Hidden Driver of Excellence. Harper.

Good Housekeeping. (2025, March 19). I'm a decluttering expert: Here are my 7 favorite methods. Good Housekeeping. https://www.goodhousekeeping.com/home/organizing/a64179214/favourite-declutter-methods/#6-the-minimalism-game

Hari, J. (2022). Stolen focus: Why you can't pay attention - and how to think deeply again. Crown Publishing.

Harris, T. (2020). The Social Dilemma [Documentary]. Netflix.

Hegedus, M. (2025, February). 9 decluttering methods that actually work. Cappuccino and Fashion. https://cappuccinoandfashion.com/decluttering-methods/

Henderson, E. & Raguse, G. (2022). Our Tried and True Tips on How to Actually Sell Your Things on Facebook Marketplace. Style by Emily Henderson. https://stylebyemilyhenderson.com/our-tried-and-true-tips-on-how-to-actually-sell-your-things-on-facebook-marketplace-even-the-best-day-to-post

Kashdan, T. B., & McKnight, P. E. (2009). Origins of purpose in life: Refining our understanding of a life well lived. Psychological Topics, 18(2), 303–316.

Ker, M. A. (2023, May 16). How to Get Your Family on Board with Decluttering. Find Your Gold Organizing Blog. https://findyourgold.ca/blog/how-to-get-your-family-on-board-with-decluttering

Lanier, J. (2018). Ten arguments for deleting your social media accounts right now. Henry Holt and Co.

Le Cras, L. (2023, March 13). 3 types of clutter you need to clear to live life lightly. Cresting the Hill. https://www.crestingthehill.com.au/2023/03/3-types-of-clutter-you-need-to-clear.html

Lembke, A. (2021). Dopamine nation: Finding balance in the age of indulgence. Dutton.

Leroy, S. (2009). Why is it so hard to do my work? The challenge of attention residue when switching between work tasks. Organizational Behavior and Human Decision Processes, 109(2), 168–181. https://doi.org/10.1016/j.obhdp.2009.04.002

Lupien, S. J., McEwen, B. S., Gunnar, M. R., & Heim, C. (2009). Effects of stress throughout the lifespan on the brain, behavior and cognition. Nature Reviews Neuroscience, 10(6), 434–445.

Mark, G., Gudith, D., & Klocke, U. (2008). The cost of interrupted work: More speed and stress. Proceedings of the SIGCHI Conference on Human Factors in Computing Systems, 107–110. https://doi.org/10.1145/1357054.1357072

Maslach, C., & Leiter, M. P. (1997). The Truth About Burnout: How Organizations Cause Personal Stress and What to Do About It. Jossey-Bass.

McEwen, B. S. (2006). Protective and damaging effects of stress mediators: Central role of the brain. Dialogues in Clinical Neuroscience, 8(4), 367–381.

Mortram, K. (2025, March 14). 10 Golden Rules for Decluttering Your Wardrobe. Good Housekeeping. https://www.goodhousekeeping.com/home/organizing/a64186053/wardrobe-decluttering-organizing-tips/

Newport, C. (2016). Deep work: Rules for focused success in a distracted world. Grand Central Publishing.

Nourishing Minimalism. (2024). How to Downsize the Kitchen: List of Necessities to Keep (Rebecca Plasters, Author). https://nourishingminimalism.com/kitchen-necessities/

Palmer, C. (2023, Oct 5). 5 Overlooked Spots You're Forgetting to Declutter in Your Living Room. The Spruce. https://www.thespruce.com/overlooked-living-room-areas-to-declutter-8768033

Pew Research Center. (2021). Social Media and Relationships. https://www.pewresearch.org/internet/2021/04/07/social-media-and-relationships/

Porges, S. W. (2011). The polyvagal theory:Neurophysiological foundations of emotions, attachment, communication, and self-regulation. W.W. Norton & Company.

Postman, N. (1985). Amusing ourselves to death: Public discourse in the age of show business. Penguin Books.

Sapolsky, R. M. (2004). Why Zebras Don't Get Ulcers. Holt Paperbacks.

Soni, P. (2023, August 28). 11 benefits of decluttering for healthy home. Amenify. https://www.amenify.com/blog/benefits-of-decluttering

Suttie, J. (2014, May 27). Why purpose is a pillar of happiness. Greater Good Magazine. https://greatergood.berkeley.edu/article/item/why_purpose_is_a_pillar_of_happiness

Sweller, J. (1988). Cognitive load during problem solving: Effects on learning. Cognitive Science, 12(2), 257–285. https://doi.org/10.1016/0364-0213(88)90023-7

Texas Commission on Environmental Quality – TCEQ. (n.d.). Household Hazardous Waste: A Guide. Retrieved 2025, from https://www.tceq.texas.gov/downloads/p2/hhw/household-hazardous-waste-guide.pdf

The Flonicles. (2023, September). The 5 types of items you should start your decluttering with. The Flonicles. https://www.theflonicles.be/en/2023/09/the-5-types-of-items-you-should-start-your-decluttering-with.html

The Spruce Editors (2023, Jan 20). 6 Tips to Be Ruthless When Decluttering Your Pantry, Organizers Say. The Spruce. https://www.thespruce.com/tips-for-being-ruthless-while-decluttering-pantry-11709626

Thomas, K. (2021, April 12). There are 5 kinds of clutter - which one is holding you back? Ideas.TED.com. https://ideas.ted.com/5-kinds-of-clutter/

Turkle, S. (2015). Reclaiming conversation: The power of talk in a digital age. Penguin Press.

Twenge, J. M., & Campbell, W. K. (2018). Associations between screen time and lower psychological well-being among children and adolescents: Evidence from a population-based study. Preventive Medicine Reports, 12, 271–283. https://doi.org/10.1016/j.pmedr.2018.10.003

West, K. (2023, Sept 8). 15 Entryway Storage Ideas to Cut the Clutter. Real Simple. https://www.realsimple.com/things-you-should-not-store-in-the-entryway-11735018

Williams, A. (2023). Decluttering Motivation Tips You Absolutely Need to Try. This Modern Mess. https://www.thismodernmess.com/decluttering-motivation-tips/

World Health Organization. (2019). Burn-out an "occupational phenomenon": International Classification of Diseases. https://www.who.int/mental_health/evidence/burn-out/en/

Zen Productivity. (n.d.). How to declutter the physical workspace by sorting and purging (step 2 of 12). Zen Productivity. https://zen-productivity.com/how-to-declutter-the-physical-workspace-by-sorting-and-purging-step-2-of-12/#:~:text=The%20process%20will%20involve%20gathering

Zuboff, S. (2019). The age of surveillance capitalism: The fight for a human future at the new frontier of power. PublicAffairs.

www.ingramcontent.com/pod-product-compliance
Lightning Source LLC
La Vergne TN
LVHW051235080426
835513LV00016B/1606